The Secret's Out!

Men and Sex, Why Women Say No

*The Perfect Guide for Women and Men
to Get the ZING Back Into
THEIR Relationships*

BY

CELIA FULLER

Social Media

Connect with me via social media:

https://www.facebook.com/pages/Celia-Fuller-Inspirational-Speaker-Spiritual-Teacher/353354161445344

http://au.linkedin.com/pub/celia-fuller/a1/7b/630

Scan this QR code with your smartphone to visit my websites,

www.wholistic-lifestyles.com.au   www.celia-fuller.com.au

Also by Celia Fuller

Kind Words Uplift

Pregnancy and Birth, The Conspiracy of Silence

The Secret's Out!
Men and Sex, Why Women Say No

The Perfect Guide for Women and Men
to Get the ZING Back Into THEIR Relationships
by Celia Fuller

ISBN: 978-0-9941518-0-3
Paintings: Celia Fuller
Graphic Art: Tamara Kempton
Typesetting: Michelle Lovi
Photos: Canstock, Shutterstock, Pixabay.

I apologize to my readers who become concerned with spelling errors. This book has been written using the American spelling as befits Amazon Publishing. If you detect spelling errors please check the different spelling versions dependent on which country you are writing from. If there remain any errors then I am happy to hear from you and will rectify any spelling that my editing team did not pick up. Thank you in advance for your care and concern.

Medical Disclaimer

At no point in reading this book should the references to products or alternative health therapists replace the need to first consult a medical practitioner.

The content of this book, *The Secret's Out! Men and Sex, Why Women Say No,* including text, graphics, images, information obtained from contributors and all other content is offered on an informational basis only. No content is intended to be a substitute for professional medical advice, diagnosis or treatment. You should always seek the advice and guidance of a qualified health provider before:

- Making any adjustment to any medication or treatment protocol you are currently using.
- Stopping any medication or treatment protocol you are currently using.
- Starting any new medication or treatment protocol, whether or not it was discussed in this book.

Information within this book is "generally informational" and not specifically applicable to any individual's medical, emotional or mental problem(s), concerns and/or needs.

If you think you might have a medical emergency, call your doctor or your local health emergency service immediately. If you choose to utilize any information provided by author Celia Fuller within the pages of *Men, Sex, and Why Women Say No,* you do so solely at your own risk.

This book might contain health and medical-related materials, which some people might find sexually explicit and personally offensive. It is the nature of this book that frank talk about, and discussions on, a variety of topics might occur. The author will attempt to moderate and review content. Purchasing, reading or digital downloading of this book constitutes acceptance of this risk.

Liability

The purchasing, reading and downloading of the book *The Secret's Out! Men and Sex, Why Women Say No,* authored by Celia Fuller, is at your own risk.

When using the material of the book, information is transmitted in ways beyond the control of the author. Celia Fuller assumes no liability for the delay, failure, interruption or corruption of any data or other information in connection with use of the digital version.

The book content of this book is provided "as is." The author, Celia Fuller, to the fullest extent permitted by law, disclaims all warranties, either express or implied, statutory or otherwise, including but not limited to the implied warranties of merchantability, non-infringement of third parties' rights, and fitness for particular purpose. Specifically, the author Celia Fuller makes no representations or warranties about the accuracy, reliability, completeness, or timeliness of the content, software, text, graphics, links, or communications provided on or through the purchasing, reading or downloading of the book.

In no event shall the author Celia Fuller or any third parties mentioned within this book be liable for any damages, including but not limited to incidental and consequential damages, personal injury, wrongful death, lost profits, damages resulting from lost data, business interruption resulting from the purchasing, reading or digital downloading based on warranty, contract, tort or any other legal theory, and whether or not the author is advised of the possibility of such damages. The author Celia Fuller is not liable for any personal injury, including death, caused by the purchasing, reading or digital downloading of this book and its content.

Indemnity

You agree to indemnify, defend, and hold harmless us, our officers, directors, employees, contractors, agents, providers, merchants, sponsors, licensors and affiliates from and against all claims, actions, demands, judgments, losses, and liabilities (including, without limitation, costs, expenses and attorneys' fees) by you or any third-party resulting or arising, directly or indirectly, out of content you submit, post to or transmit through the author's publisher, your use of this book, your connection to this book, your violation of these Terms of Use, or your violation of any rights of another person.

Acknowledgements

A special thankyou, to my husband, for his kind and considerate understanding of me, as I processed my own issues throughout our relationship. He listened to me as I explained to him how women think and feel. He is indeed an extremely patient man.

To my clients who honored and trusted me with their highly personal stories, I hope I do you justice by writing this book so it helps many more men and women through the labyrinth of relationships. Thank you for encouraging me to finally write.

Special thanks to my friend, Irene, who did my typing, and to Brett, who has been on my case to stop talking and start writing for years. Thanks also to Rodney and his team, who turned up in my life with perfect timing to support my neurosis and anxiety around publishing, and both Tamara, my son's childhood friend and Helen who added some of their great artwork to this project. Lyn, who for twenty years has guided me with any IT support and graphics and believed in any project I have started on. Great appreciation to Gail, who selflessly supported me even when she was going through her own health challenges. My dear friends, (you know who you are) who took the time to listen and also to encourage me to write. Finally, last but not least, to my mum, your advice, straightforward talking and insight throughout the years have also been embedded within these pages. Thank you.

Dedication

This book has been written for many people, but the driving force to finally put pen to paper was for you, my sons. If I could gift anything to you, it would be the capacity to master the complex nature of relationships and sexuality. You might need this reservoir of accumulated knowledge in the future. I can only hope the wisdom I have gained from my own experiences and thousands of clients will give you this essential insight, so that you learn to change, adapt and improvise.

Love Mum

Contents

Foreword

Celia Fuller admits she enjoyed a rich and fulfilling sexual life before meeting her husband of 20 years. This all came to a crashing halt after she conceived her first child so early in their new relationship. Her libido dropped to an all-time low dramatically changing how she intimately related to her husband.

The shock of those body changes and lowered sexual appetite forced her to face herself and discover why she felt and reacted the way she did. Her mind no longer seemed attached to her body. She was willing, but her body was not able. Through meditation, understanding her psychology and the gift of intuitive insight, she found a path to piece the jigsaw puzzle back together again.

Celia has been an Australian wholistic lifestyle consultant, inspirational speaker, natural therapist, counselor, and meditation teacher for over 20 years. Listening to her clients became the backbone of her research. Horrified that 90 percent of women and their partners face these same, divorce-creating issues, propelled her to write this book. Celia has woven a rich and thorough exploration of human relations together in this manual.

Housewives to career-driven women and distressed, depressed men now enjoy a full passionate life, reclaiming their inner balance and becoming optimistic with renewed creativity and forward vision. Confidence has replaced fatigue and anxiety, and careers have enjoyed a vigorous new focus and drive.

Dancing to a new rhythm, like finely strung instruments, couples have found themselves living musically by finding sexual harmony within themselves and sharing that with their partners.

This is Celia Fuller's Gift to the World.

Introduction

As a natural therapist and counselor for more than twenty years, I have seen, listened to and assisted with thousands of similar-themed distressed stories of men and women struggling with their sexual lives in relationships. When I realized how common these issues were, and the distressing toll it was taking on lives, I knew that if sexual emotional misunderstandings kept going on at the rate they were, then increases in divorce and depression would continue to rise.

From men and women in their eighties, down to their twenties, no generation has been left untouched. In the older generations, these issues never saw the light of day. But fortunately, in our open and progressive society, more people are speaking out and seeking help and understanding. It is time for me to add my voice to theirs and uncover new pathways to mending the bridge between the sexes.

The most common complaints in my clinic rooms range from women wanting natural sexual performance tablets, anxiety about fearing they don't love their partner/husband due to low sexual drive and interest, grief that their bodies have betrayed them when in their mind and heart they still want the sexual intimate connections to happen, grief and anger that their partner is becoming progressively disconnected and incommunicative, confusion about their lack of sexual interest with a partner but turned on by fantasy feelings toward others, and anger and grief about the belief that they are being treated like a nonperson.

Men come in to discuss being distressed at the lack of sex, fear that their partner does not love them anymore, anger at being made to feel rejected and not being good enough, jealousy and resentment about babies and children, fear of temptation overcoming their minds, massive levels of stress buildup due to sperm needing release and not wanting to betray the relationship, confusion about why women dress up to go out and attract other men when they don't like or want sex, and anger at feeling discarded, not important any more, used up, no joy, hen-pecked and emasculated.

So, therefore, this book has been compiled for all those men and women who are struggling with the changing nature of sexuality in their relationships and most commonly after childbirth or within a long-term relationship, with or without children.

<u>I gift this book to you.</u>

{ 1 }
Love Language of Men and Women

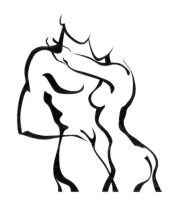

Men and women are different from one another in the way they experience life, intimacy and sexuality. Progression through life and the different phases we navigate all have an impact on our sense of personal, individual identity. Sexuality makes up a core component of how we express ourselves and connect intimately with others. Through each phase of life we change and so do our sexual appetites. To improve relationships and create deeper harmony it is imperative that we understand each other's love language. I have begun this book with a large focus on the dramatic changes that occur after the arrival of children. For my readers who are well past child bearing years you might perhaps think this section is irrelevant to your current needs, however I believe it is paramount background knowledge in helping each couple trace back where the first pain points began unfolding in their past or current relationships.

Genetically Encoded to Mate

Men and women's sexuality presents quite differently in relation to one another later in life, but not so much in the younger years. In the early developing years, hormones drive men and women to explore their sexuality in passionate demanding ways with a sense of animal urgency. Youth and new couplings feel the thrill of lust, connections and explorations. Highs experienced become intoxicating and addictive. The human body is alive and hungry from the waist down!

For years, people will experience their sexual encounters to this thrilling degree, but what happens when the thrill normalizes or changes and no longer feels new, alive and loving? Or one partner changes their reactions and perspective to intimacy but the other does not? This unevenness in relating to one another becomes a common theme of distress with the potentiality to combust into ruins. So let's examine what's going on for males and females.

In the teen years when hormones kick in and the erogenous centers become alive, the driving force to mate and procreate is the same as the animal kingdom. The biological animal side of men is programmed through deoxyribonucleic acid (DNA) to be responsible for the continuance of the species. They sow the seed, their sexual urges rarely dissipate and mental images or smells of females in need, flood their brains, often removing the capacity for normal rational thought. Even though they successfully mate, they are ready to go again and again, and any partner will do. On the emotional side, the deeply sensitive and strong emotions confuse and scare them, so they bury these deeper feelings under the urge of the sexual act. Their sexual life is rational and practical. If the need arises, fix it with the release.

Females have embedded in their DNA the need to mate, then nurture and grow the offspring to ensure the successful survival of the species. They also have an innate physical need to mate and procreate, but once pregnancy is noted in the body, the job is done. There is no more need to keep mating until their next fertile cycle comes along. This next fertile cycle occurs after birth. However the difference is, a human female's sexual encounter requires an emotional connection to feel secure that her chosen mate/partner will continue with love and support to build the nest and help with nurturing the young. The female can be turned on visually, but another more significant requirement arises—emotional connection. So even though in the younger years, wild uncomplicated sex often happens, it doesn't take long for the female to change and want more than just sex.

I know this sounds animalistic, but we're actually biological creatures inhabiting the earth with our own internal survival rhythms and cycles that must be acknowledged. However, we are also from a species that has a higher complex of a rational and emotional mind that sets us apart from the animal and plant kingdoms. Contrary to female misconceptions, men also have deep emotional aspects to their nature. They feel deeply and intensely. However, the difference between the sexes is the severe erratic nature of emotions makes men feel out of control. This sense of fear and uncertainty causes their mind to malfunction, creating a situation they would prefer to avoid.

So once they have experienced deep love and loss, they bury that aspect and allow the predictive sexual behavior to come forward. It feels to them more rational, black and white, no grey blurry aspects to deal with. In their error, they think women have done the same, so they believe all females' actions and intentions are readable according to their male definition and perception. They allow sex to become their safe version of expressing love and believe women do the same. How wrong they are and this is where the chaos begins!

Most women can certainly go hard at it, matching any man, but often it ends up being the emotional and the mental areas of loving that are the most important. It's how they learn and guarantee the survival of the young. They allow the higher nature of complex emotions to step forward and guide them, sometimes to the diminishment of practical, rational thought. The sensations of emotions help them to feel connected, alive and in touch with their surroundings. So when they couple, they need the emotional exploration to continue well past just the sex act.

Sex becomes a holistic body/spiritual experience where heaven and earth meet. When they feel that connectivity, they want to share those visions and sensations with their mate in an energetic plasma kind of way, transferring their inner beauty by osmosis, anything less than this feels selfish and not worth the effort. They fear the pain of loss, but they don't shy away from it. When these interactions are imbalanced and each partner cannot meet the other at their level, complications, hurt and resentment can arise.

Of course, not all women need the emotional encounter all the time—they can certainly embrace a good, banging, heart-pounding, sexual encounter. In fact, that is quite thrilling and intoxicating. There are also men who remain emotionally connected and are not controlled or driven by the wild untamed sexual act. Nothing is definite in our human experience, but there are a definite percentage of people I have dealt with who act and feel this way. Women want to be felt and cherished. Women believe men feel the same way. So, as you can see, there seems to be some really polar opposites in ideas and perceptions.

This is a simplistic summation of the male/female differences. As simple as it sounds, the outcome when trying to merge the sexes during long periods of time in relationships usually encounters major problems. Although society usually places relationships into the male/female-coupling category, I have also seen these same anxieties and confusions within same-sex relationships. The only difference is the same gender couplings will have the issues interspersed within one another and not always so well defined.

Pregnancy, Babies and Everything Changes

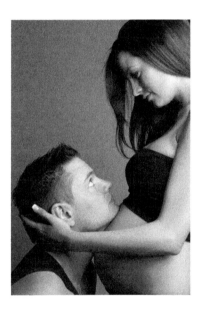

The most noted imbalances in relationships occur when the woman becomes pregnant. It is at this point that her biological need to procreate has been fulfilled, and there is no continued need to keep mating. The job is done. All her energy now turns inward to participate in the creation of new life. She is also emotionally erratic and mind numbingly exhausted. It is a rare woman who becomes highly sexed through her pregnancy. If you are a man with a wild sexualized pregnant woman in your home, then you are incredibly lucky because it is not the norm. Ninety percent of men are not getting much action at all when a woman is pregnant.

If we take our minds to the animal kingdom and study their behavior, we will find most females of the species will bite, scratch and kick the male away once they have become pregnant. Her interest will not arouse again until the birth of the babies and the fertile cycles begin. So, as you can imagine, this is the first major confusion to cross the path of the couple. The woman is excruciatingly tired and can't think properly, needing only to curl up in a ball to incubate and be held. The male is full of life ready to go hard at it every couple of hours and show his loving! He is pushed aside, alone in misery of painful genitalia and totally confused at this new rejection. Daily he walks in circles thinking, "How can I hunt my prey?" He desperately tries to understand but as soon as the woman reaches out to be held, his mind switches focus to his desperate needs.

Month after month, he tries to hold back and not be so pushy. Month after month, the woman feels guilty and tearful that her lack of sexual interest in her partner might mean that this longed-for pregnancy has been a tragic mistake. Her guilt and fear turns inward and becomes resentful at the man trying to maneuver her into having more sex. So this dance continues for nine months, each trying to forgive and discover reasons why the female body has betrayed the relationship, each of them silently waiting for the birth to come and produce the much-awaited relief, convinced it will all get better when the baby arrives. Life will be so full of love again.

Baby Arrives and All Hell Breaks Loose

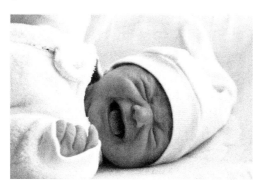

Yes, the treasured gift has arrived—a baby is born and all hell is let loose on the family home and within the intimate relationship. From day one those beautiful sensitive erogenous nipples that always used to turn the sexual passion up a notch, have now been sucked up the back of a baby's throat and mashed to pieces. Day after day, the baby devours those nipples until not a sensation ever arises from them again. The man's fun bags have been destroyed and with it the woman's loss and despair. Her body is not her own any more. She too loved the sensations of her nipple sensitivity taking her to greater heights of passion. Not any more—those GO buttons have GONE. Secretly, she hopes that it will all normalize once breastfeeding stops. Alas, the same story is told repeatedly, that those sensuous buttons are no more. A man trying to nuzzle as he has done before is more likely to be slapped aside rather than send her insides into a blissed-out sigh.

Now let's explore the lower female regions. This area after birth, has been pushed around and contorted, split, cut, torn and bruised. The female vaginal region takes quite a bit of time to repair, so again men have to do the waiting dance. They patiently wait for their favorite playground to reopen for business. For some women who are cut and torn, it can take years for the scar tissue to become less sensitive. Not only can it remain sensitive, but irregular penile angles and positioning can cause searing pain that in turn creates female aversion. Before the woman knows what's happened, her genitalia moisture has been sucked back up and the playground is suddenly closed for business, leaving the partner lost and confused at what just happened.

The woman has no language to explain, for she barely knows why she closed shop and rejected her man who has been patiently waiting all those months for a good turn with intimacy. If she does understand what has happened, she can be fearful to speak to her partner in case he feels criticized, rejected and wounded, thus complicating all the raging doubts and fears that might have already presented. A cycle of anxiety in the woman might begin at this point around her new after-baby body and how the face of the relationship has changed.

Now apart from complications in response to scar tissue, there can also be the initial lack of vaginal strength and tension—a loosened fit can remove some of the friction stimulating factors during sex for both the male and the female. This is one area that could be the seat of much anxiety and sexual dissatisfaction. Over time, with pelvic floor muscle exercises tightening can occur. A woman must be diligent to get the best effect. Who has the time for that when you have a newborn and a family to manage? It doesn't usually get done.

If all that is not depressing enough, then the G-spot can move position due to the birth changing some of the upper vaginal area. In fact, the lucky women who have never experienced an orgasm and suddenly do have been gifted with the G-spot moving into a more accessible area and easily stimulated. The men then benefit and become lucky in love. Other women who have always enjoyed that orgasmic sensation might feel it totally eludes them, as the spot has become drawn upward away from the friction of the incoming penis. They might think and secretly fear in their minds that they are no longer turned on to great heights by their partner, worrying insanely that perhaps they have fallen out of love and they are with the wrong partner. Women thinking and feeling this way could well become susceptible to postnatal depression.

Having children can really complicate this aspect of life. The saddest thing is this: all the women who come through my door feel this confusion and sadness about their body changes and the secret belief they are the only women experiencing these feelings. They walk through life in sadness and stress, constantly worrying about how they can keep their partner happy even when their own enjoyment levels aren't at their highest.

All the men I speak to think that they are the only ones feeling rejected and not getting their needs met. Yes, many men make jokes and random comments to one another, but don't actually talk and discuss it seriously to realize it is a pandemic of experience they are all transitioning through. They are all missing out.

Repair After Birth—Still No Sex

Even after most of the vagina heals, there is still no sex. By now, the woman's life has been turned upside down. Every waking moment of every day and even in the sleep state, women's minds are on guard and alert to every need of the baby. They are programmed to ensure the survival of the species at all costs and must nurture, support, feed, watch and develop their young, so the baby can finally survive on its own. This task is all consuming. It sucks up every living, breathing, remaining energy and mind attention to do this.

The baby is literally sucking the life force from your bones every time it suckles from the breast. Complex energy pathways all coordinate together to create the elixir of life-giving milk. It's exhausting, not to mention the amount of time it can take to actually get the job done. To add to this, there is the ever-present need to keep a household running and a partner fed. The baby screams, hollers and moans in pain. There are, of course, many moments that are beautiful, filled with the joy of parenting. What is so often not understood by the male is just how, all mind-consuming, looking after a child is. Not one moment in your day can be called your own as a mother. Even when the child sleeps and you sleep; it is all just to replenish the food stock of the walking, talking milk shop.

So when the man comes in the door excited to see his new family and he's faced with a red-faced woman and a screaming child thrust into his arms, it is not the time to have amorous thoughts. It is also not the time to have passing remarks about what they have done all day. This is easily interpreted by the woman as a total criticism of clothes, toys and dishes not quite put out of sight. The woman is already feeling incredibly useless and guilt-ridden that she has not performed the mother and home coordination as a superwoman would. They are usually their own worst self-critics, so if a man makes a comment, he becomes enemy number one. This scenario does not hold much hope for the man later in the night hoping for sex.

It's the Child's Fault

So day after day, the pressure of a new family member re-enacts the same sequence of events. The man facing the ever-present reality of rejection or the woman feeling resentment that she also must tend to a man's needs when her own needs don't match his. With resignation she gets the job done, or with anger, she rejects and avoids. Sometimes the woman will begin lovemaking uninterested once some build up occurs the interest can be piqued, but then usually the man who has held on for so long, has released and slumped soundly asleep without even holding the woman in the comfort and reassurance she needs so badly at this time.

Month after grueling month, with some lovely infrequent times in between, this story unfolds often without the partners really communicating their concerns. In the silence, all the man knows is that his life has drastically changed. His woman is not his woman any more, he must share her with the little creature called "child." He has to watch on as the baby has focused joy and full access to a glorious full breast. This child has usurped his number one place in the home. Every distracted moment of the day's planning is all about the baby. By the time the partner rests, she is flaked out sleeping by his side or still up when finally he gives up and sleep overtakes him. In between all that, she has turned into a snappy, bossy, control freak who just knows what a baby needs, and she thinks that he has no idea and never lets him forget it. She constantly rejects his offer of love and connection through the sexual act, as a result a nagging fear can creep into a man's mind. *Maybe she doesn't love me anymore.* And that makes the man feel angry.

Emotional Withdrawal

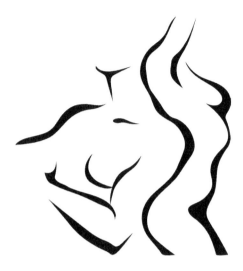

Deeply hurt by this change of lifestyle and female attitude, the man begins to retreat safely to his cave. He becomes less mentally and emotionally present, subconsciously blaming the child. He might become disenchanted with parenting or, if he feels no blame, he will just run and hide. Every attempt to create connection is faced with boredom, hostility, avoidance or rejection. For the man who needs a calm life with low emotional stress, this rapidly deteriorating scene has him running to find shelter and lick his wounds. His sexual advances lessen in frequency, too scared to face rejection again. He must keep himself safe.

The woman, although she rejects the advances, is still reeling from shock that her body is rejecting and avoiding those loving gestures. Her mind wants sex and the love life to be the same as it was before the baby but the body is defying that need. When the man stops showing his advances, either from pure understanding or not forcing the issue, or from hurt or rejection, the woman is then triggered with insecure bouts of anxiety. She might think, *Is he having an affair? He does not find me attractive. He doesn't love me anymore.* This creates a combustible fuel of anger aimed at him who dares to withdraw from the relationship when she can't ever escape, now that she has a child. She loves the child, he says he loves them all, but now he's not even trying to show any affection. Here is the moment where the man cannot win. The saying goes, "You're damned if you do and damned if you don't." The woman goes around in circles and a cycle of home craziness ensues. The angrier and more resentful she becomes, the more she says no.

How do I know this? It happened to me too!

Women Love in Multiple Ways

The language of love for women is multiple and often thought of as complex but really it's more simple than a man realizes. A woman loves by gentle affection, by listening to the thoughts and feelings of others, and she shows just how committed she is by remembering important details of another's concerns. Women do helpful acts even when not asked, just to make a person who they love, life better and easier. They cuddle and hold, offering reassurance, and stroke to soothe away the stress of life. In moments of great difficulty, they will step forward, take over and tell a loved one to rest. They talk, laugh and listen. They share the best of everything they have with another. The best of food, the biggest serving, they save the most delicious leftovers and offer them rather than eat them.

Women will listen to their partner's interests and spend hours pondering, researching and shopping trying to find the most perfect gift. All of her actions say, "I love and cherish you. Everything about your interests I have heard and I'm constantly trying to understand you and show you how important you are. I do this by reflecting back to you the purchase of gifts that say I know the things you love doing, because I heard you speak about them.

Here is a representation in gift form of your individual identity, not always something that is practical or an object you need."

The love flows in the twinkling eyes of pride, in saying thank you, in smiling in adoration, in going to events or hanging out with the partner's friends, who they are not interested in, but go anyway just to say I support your need to be your individual self. The ultimate love act is to bring a child into the world, then there is sex, and often in that order.

Women, Kids and Long Term Relationships

Before a child and when in the throes of new and exciting love, sex is often at the top of the list. It's hot, heavy, impulsive, glorious and unfettered wildness, and a discovery of newness. Every touch of a man's hand creates heat and desire, urgency to consummate as quickly and as demanding as possible. Every position, every random place is even more exciting. The man feels a woman's internal fantasies and she can meet them act for act. She is addicted to this unfettered act of loving, just as a man is. They meet equally.

After the birth of a baby, something changes from the depths of the woman. The pure intoxicating sexual act no longer delivers the fulfillment she once felt. A desperate need to be understood, supported and loved in new ways creep into her mind. Most of the erogenous buttons that once caused insane sexual delight no longer work. A woman grieves profoundly for this loss. She begins her loving language through all those other ways previously mentioned. They take precedence over the total sexual lustful act. Her sexual loving moves to a deeper, intimate, spiritual dimension of what could be called whole loving, not just genital loving. She yearns to share the core of her being, not just the external physical aspects. So a need arises where the man must identify her need to love holistically with connected, emotional understanding. The orgasm is not the end result sought; instead the lingering of love-making connection becomes the elixir. To be held and cherished with no personal expectation of needs being met is often enough and completely satisfying for a woman.

For the man, he has no idea what changed or how it changed, only that he has become an unwilling victim of that change. Now he has become caught in a whirl of elongated foreplay that is tiring with the genital pressure rarely able to withstand the onslaught of time and temptation to release. Repetitive strain injury (RSI) of many muscle groups overworked can certainly take the thrilling edge off sex. Yet the woman needs more connection for orgasm. The man's error is often the idea that a woman must orgasm every single time for her to have stress relief and feel the relationship is ok. In actual fact, being held, stroked and listened to is the new form of sexual orgasmic joy. It all spells connection and loving-ness. When the man doesn't understand this, but collapses asleep after his fun, the overwhelming sense of despondency and emotional abandonment takes hold of the female mind. She can lie for hours reviewing all that went on and her anger builds. She can feel used, abused, made to feel like a non-person, just an object used for personal pleasure and fun.

Irritatingly, the female body just begins to wake up after all the foreplay, and after the man's plunging rhythmic release, she's left on a high with nowhere to go while he is snoring next to her. She sadly climbs out of bed and completes the ironing.

Mystified at how her life experiences have gone so wrong, and are now so far removed from how she thought they would be, grief and depression could find a permanent home in her life, if the couple is not careful.

Women Have Sex by Talking

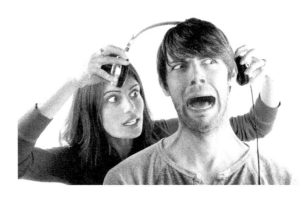

Talk with and listen to a woman and you are halfway through foreplay, especially if you are her partner! She has events throughout her day that she needs to update you on so she feels you understand her at her core and you see all the elements of her day that have molded her into the woman you discover when you come home from a day's work. Every day throughout her life, she is changing and needs you to be kept updated. She also needs to know what you feel and think so she can be reassured that you are both kept updated to the many changing perspectives and perceptions that occur during a lifetime. If this information is not fed into her circuitry, she feels disconnected, alone, irrelevant and can begin to question her existence in relation to the man.

She uses all of this inside information about a partner's feelings to orchestrate kind acts, gift giving, holiday plans, outings or adjusting her own needs to allow the man some space for him to fulfill his needs. This information also will be used in her storehouse to protect her husband from others who might insinuate negative judgments about him. She becomes his lawyer, police officer, security guard, and mother protector if the need arises and reacts according to what level of emotional mental needs she knows her man is functioning at.

This might not be a man's idea of a turn-on, but it is a woman's way of interacting. So men, if you can practice meeting her at her level more often, then your male needs for loving will become more frequent.

Men Love by Sex and Support by Solutions

The greatest confusion for women is understanding that men show their love to their partner by having sex with them and definitely not by talking. A man actually showing desire and being turned on by his partner is an outward statement of his love. Men's capacity to allow their emotions to go deeper and show their vulnerability has long been buried to keep themselves safe. Now of course, this is not the exact story for all men, but there is a majority of men who will absolutely agree with these statements. Men show their love by having sex. It's as simple and as straightforward as that.

If a woman rejects a man's advances, then it is rejecting him. It becomes personal. When he feels hurt to the core, he avoids such hurt in the future. A sexual advance in the context of a committed relationship is revealing just how invested the couple is in the relationship, especially at obvious risk of rebuttal. The male mind as mentioned earlier, is consumed by thoughts of sex—his mind continually conjures up images of sex. When men are near their partners, who have allowed them safe passage once before, their visual centers become more alive. Every action the woman makes, every body movement, is converted in their minds as a visual signal to excite and welcome sexual advances. Tantalizing images and feelings torment the male mind continuously.

During all this focused attention, the woman rarely realizes what is being plotted and planned. She is so busy that there is no awareness that she has become the target of insatiable scrutiny and fantasy. If a woman should dare approach her man with the intention to cuddle or hug, his man hormones will reach into overdrive and his body parts will immediately gear themselves up to reach the finish line, skipping all the important parts in between, unaware their behavior has suddenly become transparent and predictable when the butt squeeze enters the game.

Women are unaware of the complete intensity of thoughts that are invested with sex within the male mind. As women, they are blissfully blind to those inner taunts, as their minds do not act the same way. Yes, thoughts of sex do arise, but they are most often associated with a whole body loving, where the partner meets them emotionally and mentally as equals and in support of each other. A female's mind, in turn, goes to all those other ways of loving, and sex becomes the lovely icing on the cake.

If women truly understood the tormented minds of men, then they might actually adjust their behavior to support the men more as they try to overcome these hot and heavy urges. In those brief moments between each sexual thought, a man can then only really focus on creating solutions to problems as he deals with his day-to-day issues. For the men to have to actually slow their minds enough to follow a female conversation about all the events in the day, all the convoluted emotional issues a woman faces, just becomes impossible. Sometimes, taking the sexual pressure off the man before talking, might give him greater success, as long as it is not just before bed, because then you will be guaranteed that the whole rolling-over, sleeping scenario will ensue. It would be a great de-stressor for the man if the woman offered that to him before dinner, because then he might even listen to her. "Not likely," I hear you say. I know, but it's worth pondering just to see if the odd moment comes your way.

Different Brain Functions

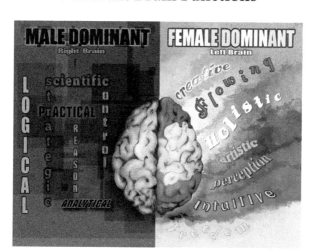

Men function primarily from a left-brain dominant attitude. This means they use their left brain in most daily interactions. If there is a problem, they fix it. They think in sequences of cause and effect and work really well within those parameters. Everything is orderly, rational and fixable. They revel in their ability to view the problem and approach it with their critical thinking. If that doesn't happen, then they read the instruction manual. Hopefully this book will become part of their essential training guide in understanding women a little better.

I often tell men, "Don't try to understand women, as they don't even understand themselves." Women sometimes have the disadvantage of being more right-brain dominant, which tends to lead them to see the biggest wholistic picture of a problem or situation and take all the convoluted paths to discover the solution. This could be seen as dithering and unfocused, but in truth women operate from an experiential formula. They see and feel from other people's points of view and also their own. They gently navigate to find a solution that fits well with all concerned.

This behavior model can cause them to become too entwined

in an issue and then not be able to make decisions to rectify it. When a woman tries to find an immediate solution in the relationship to keep the man happy, she will usually pluck the first thought she has out of thin air. But this doesn't mean the comment is really based on truth, because she has not had enough time to sit and ponder or talk it over and then talk some more.

So when major communication occurs, it is often the woman who has not yet found the true cause of her discontent but keeps dragging up the past, saying it's this, or it's that, but in truth, it's neither. It could be the truth is so personal and hurtful to her partner that the words just will not come out! She will harbor the words for longer in the hope the man will become an instant mind reader overnight and then no explanation will be necessary. Or she might hope that it will be easier to speak out the next time.

When men feel personally attacked from comments about the bedroom antics and the way they show love, they become mortally wounded and clam up and stop communicating. They can withdraw emotionally and be less interactive. This behavior confirms to the woman why she never spoke up before. When a man clams up emotionally, it's even harder for a woman to have intimacy. She also falls into a wounded silence. This state creates extra fears resulting in her building a new arsenal of behaviors against the man and makes it that much harder to find the real reason behind her emotional woes and discontent.

A loop of stress begins—the man needs more sex and release. He needs reassurance of loving so that his kind of loving becomes the healing balm. The woman needs to talk more and try to explain herself out of feeling guilty as her healing balm, while the man is driven even more mental. Someone has to take the leadership role and it's usually the woman.

Men Love to Get the Job Done

A surefire way of helping a man feel you understand him is meeting him at his level. The need for sexual release is paramount for his brain to operate properly without short-circuiting and to feel loved and appreciated. If his needs are met, the emotional wall of non-communication will gently lower, and he'll become more interested in the woman's world because she came into his.

Many women faultily believe they are deceiving the man if they do not offer a full body sexual vaginal encounter with all the emotional trappings that go with it. This is because this is how a woman would feel with her own chosen intimacy. She wants the whole deal. Anything less is a rip-off. Men, on the other hand, love uncomplicated sex, where he does not have to think, plan or be always considerate. He wants full-blown visual cues and a good firm grasp in the genitalia. They are more than happy for the woman to give them a good robust hand job or fellatio, or even just use her body parts to rub up against. It's a huge turn-on if they don't have to be considerate. All they want is to go for it. It's even better if the woman offers her services tending to his every need like a king. This is why the pornography and prostitution industries are so appealing. They don't have to care about how a woman feels.

The men get so turned on because their minds can become fully immersed in the act that they so hunger for. They mostly do not mind missing a fully connected intimate lovemaking session. It takes too long! Sadly, this is where the male and female species diverge so much. Women are sure they want some of the action but feel guilty if they don't provide it.

This book is for you, ladies—you can take the pressure off yourself and the relationship. You can give your man many more intervals of his needs being met without your whole body being invaded. If you can find the energy and time just for him to get his release, then you have also gifted yourself some time for your own sexual rhythms to catch up and be ready to enjoy a full lovemaking session where your body is turned on more easily because the partner is happier and nice to you. In addition, your body has had time to allow the urgency feelings and hormonal changes to trigger a bigger interest in sex. It will also take the pressure off you, when in the past you had to lay there waiting for him to fumble around, become insanely aroused and two minutes later be finished. A few extra hand jobs between good lovemaking sessions will help him become more adaptable and have endurance and self-control. This is good for both of you.

Now I realize this is not always easy for women to actually step up and give him what he wants, yet again without you having any joy in return. It's worth a try just in case your relationship becomes empowered by this. If, however, you still think giving fellatio or a hand job is an invasion of your personal space and personal being, then I certainly don't advocate that you force yourself to serve him and then feel used, abused, dirty or stained as the outcome. This is unhealthy for both of you. Only offer when you know it feels emotionally and mentally safe to do so. Above all, you must learn to communicate.

Men, you must gently explain, encourage and reassure your partner that you would be happy for them to oblige you by offering some form of uncomplicated emotional lovemaking sexual favor. A woman is usually desperate to please her mate, so reassurance will really help. Women do not automatically know this about men, because they experience loving so differently. As a special note, women, please don't spoil your men with this option too often, otherwise he can become lazy and selfish in relation to your needs being considered. This works both ways.

CAUTION! I must mention here that for a man to have to maintain a hard erection through hours of foreplay to help a woman have an orgasm or be turned on at all is not possible. It might have been that way when he was younger, but as the years slip by it becomes more difficult to "keep it up." Remember, it is blood flooding to the penis muscle that keeps the firmness. This blood rushes in when there is the sense of sexual desire that might become satisfied. If that urge is activated, but then held back for large periods of time to pleasure their partner, then there will be a diminishment of the erection with the risk that a woman will think she is not desirable. She was, but the man's mind became sleepy and the urgency switched off. It is not personal; it is just a fact about how the man's anatomy works.

Grope, Grab, Twist and Turn

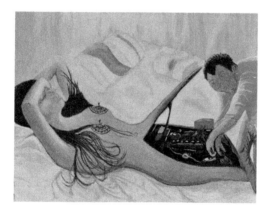

What is going on? Has my lover turned into a car mechanic overnight?

Have you lost your minds, men? What are you thinking when you attack every sensitive tissue on the female body with a series of twists, honks, pulls, contorts and clit banging as though you are working under the bonnet of a car? Has the lady lost her face? Have you forgotten she even has an upper body? Or, is your toy broken and you are desperately trying to fix it? Well, STOP IT! Have you ever noticed that when the women is moist and wanting more action that your tweaks, grabs and pokes cause a groan of distress and she dries up and the legs begin to close. That's right! Those groans are not always of pleasure. If you notice she dries up, then you probably hit a sensitive spot and she is over it for the night. It takes a lot to awaken her sexual appetite but not much to turn it off.

Hers is a modern engine with all the fine electrical wiring and delicate sensors. Yes, that's right, tricky stuff. Not many mechanics know how to play in that playground. COMMUNICATE. Ask what you did wrong. Ask the woman to show you how it could be done better. Her response might be a frustrated "Oh, it doesn't matter!" Hrrrmph. Don't believe her. IT DOES! So don't keep proceeding to get your rocks off. Slow down, speak gently to her and begin a new touch. If you don't, you will end up paying for it.

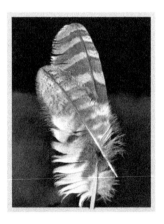

Instead imagine you are an expert archaeologist.

That's right! I have given you a female hint. If you are not sure what that looks like or what they do, GO TO YouTube. There is usually a feather, soft blowing actions and gentle tender finger motions as they slowly uncover an ancient artifact of great value. If you can't imagine that, then think of a beautiful flower that has come into blossom. The petals are open. Now, do you snatch, grab, pull and contort the petals? NO! So, STOP IT. You are NOT a mechanic (some of you might be). YOU ARE A LOVER! Learn to love differently.

On the other hand, **women, you need to become race car drivers** and great car mechanics. Grab hold of that stick. The boys love it. Stand aside and they will show you how. Then practice, and practice some more. Men are patient while you learn and they are even happy to assist. Become a team and use teamwork.

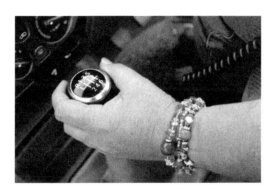

Now here's the next question to be asked, When can the man stop being an archaeologist and get down to serious men's business?

Well, this is where observant body reading enters the game. You will have to step up, watch, listen, feel and become almost a mind reader. This is only a general guide because all women's body needs are different. So here we go with some graphic visuals.

As you explore the vaginal regions delicately and you notice moisture formation, then this is the beginning of the automatic body reaction readying the woman for penis entry. Now I say it is getting ready, but don't begin madly plunging nonstop! The moisture actually has a slightly numbing aspect to it and magically enhances the tissue sensitivity, making those finger moves even more intoxicating. Increased finger probing to greater depths will usually have the woman begin to pelvic rock a little with her body warming to you. If she pelvic rocks, or if light murmuring sounds escape, they are all good signs that your wait is nearly over. Teasing her with the penis head just within the opening or moving it up and down from clitoris to vagina to clitoris again can also speed the process up.

When her rocking becomes stronger and rhythmic, then go for a plunge and see what the reactions are. Don't go hammering violently straight up. Go hard a few times then tease again until she is demanding it, then go hard again. Fast, fast, slow, slow, drawn out to the point that you are almost pulled out as though giving a nonverbal threat that you are going to stop. At some point, she will either start grabbing your butt or leg to facilitate deep thrusting or you will have gone to the place of no return. As you perfect this and you observe all the different heights your partner and you can reach, you will also develop the skill of holding out for longer.

Alternatively, you can remain fully penetrated with no movement and allow for only the small muscular flexing moves of the penis. Do not underestimate the power of not moving within the woman. For the woman, internal sensation of parts of her anatomy will feel like they are opening up and wrapping around the penis, literally making way for even deeper, gentle penetration and soul-satisfying, whole-body climaxes.

Then begin your serious men's business for the finale!

Remember erogenous zones of the woman cannot be attacked and groped. They need tenderness, nibbling and nuzzling.

Extra Helpful Hints

Kissing—Most importantly you need to know a woman's whole body is a sexual organ, not just her clitoris or vagina. Kissing and neck nuzzling is vitally important and a step that should not be overlooked. By the gentleness of a kiss on the forehead, over the face and then fully into the mouth with increased fervor you are already hinting at the pleasure you want to give as you progress through other parts of her body. Treat her face, jaw, neck and mouth as though it is a reflection of her lower anatomy and you will notice that her lower half begins to respond even without you touching it. The way is preparing itself for your entry. The combination of tenderness and urgency ensures a woman feels you have honored her as a person and desire to know her fully, not just as a vagina with a head attached.

Kiss, Lick, Nibble and Stroke the Whole Body—Now I know this takes time but it is worth the effort and if you, as the man, let the woman fully treat your body in the same way, you might be pleasantly surprised how deep your own lovemaking experience can go.

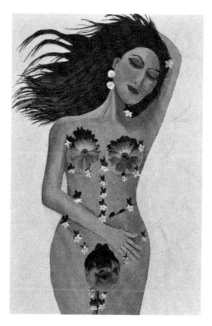

This process should be done slowly, but at times, the energy can demand that everything speeds up. Again, combinations of fast devouring and slow lingering can really get those juices flowing. As you slowly make your way down the body, be aware that every gentle hand/finger stroking movement is literally turning the fire up. A female's skin is extremely sensitive to this excitement. Trace around the fullness of the breasts, do not grab and pull the nipple straight away. Each area must be awakened before you go for the grab or nibble.

Don't overlook the crease in the elbows, under the arm, curve of the lower back toward the buttocks and even behind the knees and feet. The inner thighs should be stroked with gliding movements, just ever so tantalizing touching the labia as they pass through, progressively treating her vagina and clitoris like an archaeologist would touch a delicate flower. Eventually you begin a more in-depth exploration of her intimate zone, however, never forgetting she still has the rest of her body and feelings. So it's always good to leave the playground from time to time by way of kissing and stroking the other parts of her body. This way you are saying, "All your body excites me, and I long to know it all."

Men Don't Always Want Sex, They Do It FOR YOU!

Ladies, this might come as surprise to you, but there are actually times in a relationship that a man might not feel like sex, contrary to popular belief. You might not know this because he will actually put his own feelings aside (just like women often do) and instigate lovemaking because he believes it will make the woman feel nice and less agitated. (*It works for them, why not for the woman?*) Sadly, when they do this, especially after a fight or argument, the woman goes into a hurtful inner rage or negative dialogue, thinking the man is using sex to apologize (sometimes they are) or assuming sex will make the issue go away. Some women will even go as far to think that his behavior of follow-up sex confirms her negative thinking that she is just a body with no brain, no feelings and there he goes again chasing his own needs without thought for his partner that he professes to love. It's all about *him*. Sometimes a female's mind is her worst enemy with inner assumptions and contorted perceptions.

While a woman is thinking these thoughts about the man, he is on the surface looking as if he has had a great time and then he falls soundly asleep. HOWEVER, he also has an inner dialogue where he really has to work hard to keep an erection and follow through with attempted pleasuring to be the soothing balm to his partner. All the time really feeling, not that into it, but happy enough to show support and be present for the partner and ease whatever distress is happening.

A man might feel this way due to situations at work or in the home environment, which might have triggered the man to become deeply emotionally hurt, rejected or criticized. Sometimes men might even switch off their wish for intimacy through being involved in deeply emotional situations or watching sensitive material on television or movies. When these feelings arise, he is personally struggling to get a grip on his own inner turmoil of self-doubt and negative talk. It is at this time he might be inclined to just roll over and avoid making love.

If, however, the woman begins to stroke him caringly for no other reason than to show love and support, the man might presume she is angling for more action and, through guilt at his withdrawn state, he gathers himself to give her a good time, even when it never was on her agenda.

WORST CASE SCENARIO: the woman's stroking is misinterpreted, she did not want sex (just a cuddle), but now she is also having sex out of guilt because she does not want to reject his loving advances.

Around and around we go in these non-talking, non-communicating scenarios void of open and frank honesty. If a man explained that he did not feel like having sex because he feels off, then the woman instead of quietly accepting and just being gentle and kind will want to TALK to him about it. Her own fear that she is the cause of his inner distress will propel her to interrogate him. From a man's viewpoint, it is just easier to not talk about it. It's a lot more peaceful. What to do? LISTEN or be silent. Don't TALK.

My husband cannot even think about making love if he has watched a deeply emotional film. It stirs up his sensitive side and he needs time to allow the thoughts, material and images to settle in his mind and ponder on. Of course, for me, being female, this is exactly when I do wish to connect in such a deep and sensitive way. Imagine the confusion I felt when I would be faced with lovemaking avoidance or outright rejection when I instigated wanting sex. I now know if I want ACTION, then I have to avoid such films. On the positive side, I am grateful that he actually is affected by emotional sensitive movies and by the content. This brings him closer to me in so many other ways. My Solution: avoid all sensitive media and find a new playground.

I share this story because our men are more complex and deeply thinking and feeling than we often give them credit for. We need to take time to understand them more by deep observation, because we can't actually ask because that's talking about ***feelings.***

{ 2 }
Helpful Hints for Men
to Get More Action

Create Safe Intimate Spaces without Expectation

Men, here is a list of some helpful tips for you, so it makes your journey easier and women also get their needs met. I hope the women reading this book will devour every word and open up an honest dialogue with their partners about some of these thoughts and ideas. Men need guiding in these delicate matters. This is where same-sex couples, especially female couples, have an upper edge because they understand more closely how they feel in relation to their body and communicate openly and often effectively. Heterosexual women get all caught up in themselves, expecting the men to be mind readers and they find it hard to explain why some behaviors are detrimental to the positive growth of the relationship. Ladies, in the end it is up to you to help the partner in your life know how to navigate the complexity of your emotional states and your physical bodies.

Flowers, a Gift of Guilt or Love?

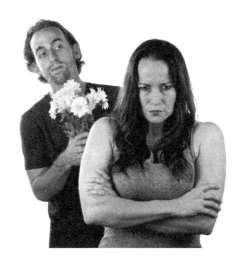

Sometimes men overdo the gift of flowers or give them at the wrong time. Marketing and TV shows tell them that this is what women want. They are also told that gifting of flowers will gain them instant forgiveness and fix any wrongs that have occurred. They have been led to believe that flowers are the winning formula for making up after ugly fights and damaging words. This, however, is not the truth. Yes, many women do love flowers, as they are delicate like we are, but when they arrive constantly after a fight and there is no change in future behavior, they lose their healing balm and only become an agitation. If flowers arrive mysteriously followed by a guilty look on a man's face, then there will be more questions surrounding the gift. However, beautiful spontaneous flowers can really create a new connection of loving, especially if the man has added his own words in a card, revealing he has made an extra deep thinking effort—not just a grab and run fix. We are forgiving and lenient, so even a grab and run can have a positive effect.

What Flowers Can't Do, But a Man Can!

Sadly, flowers can't wash the dishes, vacuum the house, do the ironing or clean the oven, bathroom or toilet. They can't make the lunches, feed the pets, make and serve dinner, replenish the beer or cup of tea, clean the sheets, chase perpetual washing all over the house, fold the clothes, pack the clothes away and do the shopping. They can't be called on to be a taxi for all the family, speak to schoolteachers, help with homework and tutoring, give a massage, give one hour of free time for a women to emotionally prepare for sex, take a screaming baby for a walk or drive, care for aging parents or wake up through the night soothing a stressed child.

Gifting flowers can, however, bring a smile to the face and warmth to the heart encouraging a woman to keep going. However with a generous, thoughtful helping hand to lighten your partner's workload, an alternative path to better relations and less resentment might appear.

Household Responsibilities Destroy Sex!

Did you know that many women learn to loathe cooking? Imagine that during a lifetime, a woman is expected to cook night after night and provide meals and lunches for all the times in between. By the time a woman hits menopause, she is OVER IT! Many elderly men in counseling are shocked at this because they have been brought up with the TV showing them that women love to cook! It would seem a woman couldn't wait to tend to his every need and that of the family. Or the men have seen their mothers acting like they love it and can't wait to do more of it. Men believe that it's the only thing women talk about, so they must love it.

Well, I have news for you. Those same mothers come to me in

deep despair complaining of the never-ending cycle of cooking, washing, cleaning and caring. Their life has been sucked dry by the constant drudgery of menial work and they feel as if they have experienced life as a factory worker without any life or inspiration at the end of the tunnel.

I remember this story of a woman who had hit menopause. Her children had left home and she along with her husband were thinking of downsizing from their lovely home into something quite simple. She quietly told me that all she wanted was a house with a concrete floor. The kitchen had to have a table with metal plates bolted to the table so that when mealtime was finished, she could get the fire hose out and blast the plates dry, wash the floor and walls all in one quick session.

They were actually planning to live in a shed. Hmmm, I was only 26 when she told me that, so I laughed along with her humor. But, you know, I did note a determined, deadly serious look in her eyes behind the humorous twinkle, and I never forgot that look. Since then I have heard hundreds of that same type of sentiment, but perhaps without the extreme living circumstance as a solution. Being older now, I completely understand—but I don't have a fire hose or concrete floor.

Another common story that comes up in counseling is the caravan and motor home dream. It starts off with the woman thinking that by running away from home and finally discovering a world out there after children, she would be released from the daily tasks of cooking, cleaning and washing. Somewhere in her deluded mind, she must have thought the man would suddenly realize that he was retired and could no longer claim work fatigue from chore avoidance. In fact, he might even realize how hard she has had it all these years, and acknowledge that now they both are on equal footing to share those mundane tasks, he might actually jump in and help.

Sadly, this realization is not often the case. She works toward her dream, only to find she becomes trapped in a smaller house where she can't escape night-time snoring, channel surfing or the incessant blaring of the TV or radio, while the man sits ever so patiently for his meal to be served, then taken away and magically washed up. The woman, in the meantime, is seething with anger, resentment and quite possibly hot flushes and a dose of hurt while he wanders outside to find other men to crack open a beer with. She, and every other woman, is hanging the washing out to dry, listening to the guffawing tall stories of the men.

Now I am not in the retired demographic yet, but when I hear these stories repeatedly told to me, it really can destroy my own ideas and fantasies of the dream. Women reveal they often regret deciding to go traveling, because it has caused more disrespect for their partner. Some have refused to travel in this way anymore. For women who love to travel, usually their men have already understood this and agreed to share the chores.

So men, if she only talks about food all the time, it might be because it fills her waking moments, and in some small degree, she feels as if it's making up for the loss of sexual fun she does not provides the man with. There is a saying, "A way to a man's heart is through his stomach." Well, that is quite true, because when you cook it reminds a man of his mother's love—his first love. So the woman tries valiantly to provide for his needs, but by the time the kids have hit their early teens, she is well and truly over it. She becomes ferocious, verbal and resentful. Sex declines.

So I say to women, "Don't cook all the time!" Men are not useless—they just don't want you to know that. Children, up to a certain age, are far more capable than you might realize. Make fruit platters and soup portions that last for days and keep loads of canned goods handy. The same goes for ironing. MEN—Please speak up and keep convincing your partners to NOT DO THE

IRONING, unless they are about to go out and need something to wear, or if they absolutely love it. How many of your partners iron into the late hours of the night, only to have all those wasted hours wrecked by children dragging their pressed clothes out of the closet and leaving them in a crumpled heap on the floor? Or they iron, and then pack the clothes into crammed wardrobes, only to be wrinkled again when you pull them out? If a partner is adamant to keep ironing, then try and understand her personal perspective about the matter. Make her a cup of tea, at the very least, before retiring to bed as a form of solidarity. Show her you appreciate all her endeavors.

Ladies: Free your mind from the extra stress. Keep your energy for sex instead.

Domestic Foreplay

Women are much simpler to get around than men think they are. It does not take much attention to have her swoon with inner delight and begin the process of what might be called domestic foreplay. If your woman is washing up and you are thinking about relaxing, watching TV, enjoying a beer or a cup of tea as you might normally do, then change your habits. Have you ever thought that she might like to sit and join you? But she is too aware that the washing up has to be done and she'll be expected to do it. Well, try another tack.

Stand by her side, gently place your hand on her shoulder and ask if she needs help. What happens inside her body is amazing when you approach her with GENUINE interest. Inside her body, she'll be swooning with a heat-fluttering reaction. Relief at being noticed, a feeling of importance and even sexual heat due to the connection and understanding will rush through her and into the groin. So emotionally affected and surprised by your kind offer, she'll probably say, "No, it's ok, I can do it." So the plus side is you can still relax with the happiness knowing that you just made another person feel happy and appreciated.

She'll continue washing up, with lightness in her heart and in her step. She might just let you come near her tonight. If, on the other hand, she accepts your offer to help, then while you stand together working, a feeling of energy plasma of connectedness is forming, just like a dance. This heightened sensitivity of your nearness and attentiveness will begin to operate on those sensuous levels that men are so focused on. A woman needs to feel togetherness, a sharing of the burden being turned into joys. There is more likely a chance of tenderness later in the evening. WARNING: Don't grope or handle her at this stage or she will be onto your plan.

Walk Next to Her, Not in Front

Another effective way for a woman to feel connected and loved is by walking next to her and gently placing your hand on her lower back. Do not push her along; it makes her feel as if you are shoving, and then anger follows. Instead, place your hand gently in the small indentation of the lower back. This gesture says, "We are together and I care about you." It also shows to the world that you are committed. A woman feeds off that. Again, if done gently, she'll swoon and completely feel loved and considered. A rush of sexual energy might even be felt in her lower region. This again will help her self-confidence and connection to you. It often will ignite more interest in the relationship and provide the essential emotional link for later bedroom antics. Feelings that she has put on ice and relegated to the TOO-HARD BOX might just defrost. When a woman opens up emotionally, so do her body parts.

WARNING: DO NOT place your hand on her neck when walking! That feels as if you are controlling her and warning her that she will be strangled if she misbehaves. It's not hard to just think about the woman's needs sometimes. These might be subtle gestures, but do not underestimate their power.

Holding Hands—No Dragging

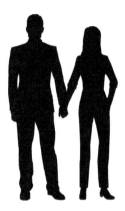

Holding hands is another lovely gesture and often gets discarded when you are both used to lugging bags, wheeling strollers and holding children. By the time you're ready to hold hands again, you've forgotten how to do it. It's important for each partner to walk at a pace that matches the other. Dragging along the foot-path or leading like a friendly pet dog does not work. Resentment and anger are the typical responses of women, to this style of handholding. You will find that your partner will not reach out as often, if this occurs on a regular basis.

Go Shopping Together

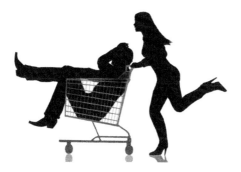

Make shopping a thing you sometimes do together, or even do it for her. The relentless task of shopping for the family is mind numbing. Battling crowds, juggling screaming children and even working out what to buy, can take the edge off any good day. When you accept that you are both in this relationship together, with all the same needs for your family, then it only stands to reason to offer your help. By this action, you are acknowledging your awareness of the pressure she is under and you are going to support her. Luckily, in this modern era, younger women are easing the burden by online shopping. Having said that they still need free time in front of the computer to put the order through. She probably is doing this late at night while you are in bed waiting for her.

Sitting Watching TV Close Together—No Groping

When sitting watching TV, allow your body language to come close to her, but no groping. Just sit and feel connected. This is not easy for a man, as his mind can't think straight or watch a show if he's cuddled up close. His anatomy and mind become agitated with other interests. If the man allows this behavior to overrule the close encounter by insisting on the groping technique of fore-play, then the woman will suspect that the only reason for sit-ting close is the easy access to her female parts, and that he is not thinking about providing a safe intimate space without scheming one of his man plots.

Bed-Hug without Sexual Advances—No Groping

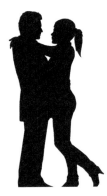

When in bed, hug sometimes without expecting the next stage of intimacy. Allow the woman to feel that you wish to comfort her and support her without needing more from her. For a woman to receive a hug without sexual prompting is the ultimate togeth-erness. It makes the day seem worthwhile, especially when there is the juggle of crazy family life or a partner is deeply involved in supporting aging parents or grieving about something. Expecting or demanding sex at a woman's high time of distress is not the correct formula of helping. That is the man's way.

If a man can make allowance for the woman's needs in this matter, his partner will feel so much more appreciated. For the man this is difficult, so men, if you need to remove yourself from the bed because the pressure inside you is too unbearable, then leave the room and relieve yourself of the pressure. Do not stay in the room or in the bed doing this, as it might be seen as a form of punishment for the woman, especially if done with anger by violently and dramatically tugging away on your own body. This behavior can invoke either guilt or disdain from the woman—not a good recipe for more things to come.

Beware of Predictable Behavior When Hugging

Make a habit when you hug or hold a woman that you keep it clean—no grabbing butt cheeks, pelvic thrusting—or groping at the breasts, either from behind or the front. If you only do these behaviors randomly, it can be quite sexy and a good laugh, but if you do it as a constant prelude to expecting more in bed later, then your behavior becomes transparent and predictable. Women will quickly be disturbed by your actions and not find them funny. They become the actions that make a woman feel like she's only valuable and useful for one thing—the man's sexual pleasure.

Men, Bedrooms Are Boring and Predictable

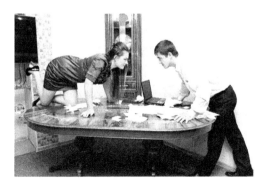

There is a danger among men toward a comfort zone of sex. Men often fall into a complacent, easy access form of sexual advance that becomes boringly predictable. As men, you might not realize just how transparent your behavior is, but to a woman your actions and intentions are obvious. So obvious, that women have developed a multitude of skills to avoid your physical and verbal cues around sex.

Women love the thrill of being chased, desired and hungered for. They want to feel that a man is so overwhelmed by the intensity of inner love that his advances toward them are spontaneous and fueled by the need to merge in emotional closeness—right here, right now, an overwhelming desire. Women are constantly in love with the feeling of being in love. They never want the feeling of first passionate love and connection to ever go away, this is their food for the soul and why romance novels are so popular. These fantasy stories describe scenes of urgent secret love that two people mutually felt and then could not hold back from expressing. These slightly erotic encounters occur rarely in the bedroom or in the cover of night. Those scenarios encapsulate the overall sentiments of women.

How many movies or TV shows have scenes with blistering, erotic, uncontrolled sexual escapades on the stairs, over desks, in the kitchen, in elevators or in plane restrooms? Where do you think they get those ideas? These are the thoughts of women's secret fantasy worlds. Women's novels are full of similar styled scenes. Why? Because it is what women want out of life. They yearn to feel so alive again.

A woman wants to be loved all over the place. Think of the house, there are more rooms than just the bedroom. Other rooms in the house are quite fine, even while washing up. I know it becomes quite impossible with children, because they always seem to tune in to your closeness and charge through the door. But even the beginning effort is fuel to the female fire. She will then more likely find a way to continue, even if in a smaller way, where you left off. If a man pouts or gets angry, especially with the children, her anger will arise to defend them. Find humor and walk away, leaving the promise in the air. Dare I say, try it outside in the night air, rekindling memories of youth and laughter away from the ears of sleeping children. Or what about in the car parked in the driveway while your teenagers take over every room in the house and tread the floorboards at night? *Dare to do it differently.*

Make excitement return to your life. Women dream about this exciting connection in almost equal portions to a man thinking about sex. I say "almost" because really the percentage in a day where a woman's mind ponders on sex is not nearly as much as the man, but it can be vastly increased with positive thoughts, not ones of insecurity, fear and avoidance.

Men, stop thinking comfort zone. If you want sex in your life, you must discover the inner hopes and dreams of your partner. As you listen to them, they will give you signals and opportunities on a constant basis. Listening, and I mean proper listening, is a turn-on and early foreplay. Talking removes the daily grind from a woman's mind, reducing her back to her original self before children. That is where a man needs his woman's mind to be.

{ 3 }
Private Thoughts of Women

In this next section I will be sharing some of the secret thoughts, concerns and anxieties women hold within the back of their minds and rarely share with their partner. Many of these examples are constant thought streams running through the female mind destroying her ability to completely relax and enjoy sexual activity.

It is hoped by sharing this information that partners might be able to allay those secrets anxieties and offer words of encouragement and support or find ways to alleviate those fears nestled within the deep recesses of the female mind.

Love, understanding and compassion go a long way in winning the hearts of women.

Bedroom Antics and Women

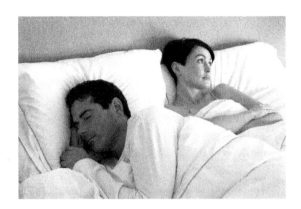

The woman knows the bedroom is her worst nightmare and emotional battleground. If she is having a huge dilemma about her sexual feelings and hoped for, but often eluded, sexual gratification, then the bedroom is a place of heightened anxiety. She fears that every night all she will be is a stress relief for a man. When the man go to bed then she runs a mile in the opposite direction, only to have to come to bed once he's soundly sleeping. Knowing there is a high chance of more adventure in the morning, she leaps out of bed earlier. She knows that when a man wakes up he has an erection, usually associated with a full bladder. Strangely though, the man with an engorged penis prefers to not waste the opportunity by emptying his bladder. Instead, he allows the pleasure signals to fill his brain and pursue fantasies of thrusting.

Men, women over time come to know the erection is just a biological reaction, not a reaction that upon opening your eyes you have become intoxicated with love for your woman and then has an urge to show undying love. She sadly comes to accept this fact and knows, at best, the man might have had an erotic dream of pursuing her in his nighttime sleep and then wakes up to continue it. More likely the nightscape is full of dreams of many different possible sexual objects, which is one more explanation for the awakening erection.

So the bedroom at night becomes synonymous with stress relief, snoring and rejection for both men and women. In the morning a biological erection devoid of initial lovingness pushes the sheets up. If a man can actually think before he acts, he can transform the mornings into a powerful opportunity to engage in true, emotionally nurturing states, with sex not always the obvious outcome. This opportunity could initiate a deeper, more fulfilling journey.

If choosing night-time sexual fulfillment, then the best time for a man or woman's sexual fulfillment is in the middle of the night when they are both rested to a degree and there is still more time ahead for deep restful sleep after the fun. If either man or woman was to wake up and approach the other in a gentle, slow, non-demanding way, showing by action the depth of lovingness, then those actions become more than physical needs. Imagine you have woken from precious sleep, to discover your partner is taking the time and care to slowly arouse your body. Waking from sleep in this manner is a surprise gift and seems to heighten all the senses making it a precious time with more chance to be received well. Many couples have found a great connection in the wee small hours between children waking, musical beds and snoring. In the middle of the night, early angers have lessened or disappeared, making way for new communications.

Women Want Sex! Don't Be Fooled, Men

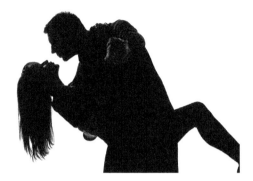

Don't be fooled men by the lack of sex you have with your partner. Do not fall in the trap of thinking that she has lost all interest in sexual activity because she no longer shows enough interest in you.

She does not hate sex, unless there are past emotional events that have damaged her in this way. Women want sex. She wants sex to be hot and heady, the end result of two people feeling the magnetic attraction of first love. She wants newness, spontaneity, non-predictability and her body treated with reverence and hot desire. She thinks about the lost days of loving lust and attraction, often yearning for that newness of connection to return. She fervently seeks for it in the eyes and actions of a partner, wanting that pulse of life to flow through her every cell. She looks to feel for that time when the man's connection to her had him speaking about his innermost thoughts and desires and he listened to hers. This is her vision of sharing his life essence and learning about how events have changed and molded him. She yearns for a sense of belonging and specialness.

With her heart desperate to awaken back to those first moments of new love she shared with her partner, she potentially becomes a victim of another man's attention. Even though a woman does not feel sexy toward her husband, she can quickly fire up the cauldron of forgotten love lust, if a new man puts in the ingredients she needs. A new man has none of the remembered predictability, bad habits, negative words, and impatience with kids, or roaming eye. Not yet anyway.

A woman can fantasize the reality out of any situation to serve her need to be taken on a mystical journey of love. So beware men, there are predators among your species, as you well know, and one of them might speak the love language of your woman. Her potential to stray hangs with how well you match that language and make her feel special. She will not take up that new offer readily or easily, but if her feelings are aroused, it could sow the seeds of doubt within her as to where her heart belongs. Remember, the new man is offering by way of feeling and connection, a window back to her former sensual, sexual self, before children and marital responsibilities. It's an intoxicating mix.

Just as with men and temptation to wander from monogamous sex, so too are women equally at risk. Neither man nor woman should let the current committed relationship dive into states of paralytic boredom, predictability and negativity. You owe it to each other to work toward maintaining the strength of communication and connectivity.

If women did not want sex or were not interested, then the statistics in the United States, revealing that one in every three women watch pornography, would not be accurate. Many also read it.

So here is a secret I will share with you. I just mentioned how women love to be loved and feel the magnetic attraction and want open communication of feelings. This is all true, especially in a committed relationship where those ingredients are vital to her. But there is more. She is also equipped with inner fantasies that she is not even properly aware of because they arise from her unconscious awareness.

Written pornographic literature, otherwise known as Literotica, knows this and uses that information to create highly addictive stories with consumer evidence indicating that this style of literature is becoming increasingly popular. In past generations there were always some soft-porn stories, but the closest novels that women could read without being accused of being low, dirty or reading smut were the famous Mills and Boon romance novels, also known as Harlequin romances. Women will confess that with the gentle erotic scenes in these books and the clever build-up of sexual tensions, the words had the power to ignite the female fantasy world and activate a solo body reaction.

This is due to a specific writing formula that has been proven to work. Literotica uses the same basic formula for writing stories that are bound to make women feel a little hot and heavy. Research has shown women's sexuality first activates at a primal level within the reptile brain, our animal self. In this part of the brain, females are programmed with an unconscious reaction hungering for what is known as the obsession storyline.

Basically, it goes something like this: The woman, often helpless or vulnerable in some aspect of her personality, creates such an impact on the man's mind that he overcomes all resistance internal and external to have her. She wants to be taken not viciously or violently, but with fervor, demanding and hungry. Desired from every pore of the man's being, right there, right now, with no delay. Consumed by the soft-skin touch, his urgency is made known to her. Effectively his demands and needs for her causes her to lose her mind and all rational thought and allows herself to be taken. At this stage, she will be more open to daringly explore her body and her partner's body. Men, do you make your women feel completely desired?

On a cautionary note, Literotica is a form of entertainment but it is highly addictive and avidly read by both men and women to provide a colorful fantasy world full of potential disappointment, because real life often does not look like that. In the beginning of a relationship it probably did. This is how we manage to couple. These fantasy excursions can create high relationship expectations, not matching reality. Sadly for a woman, once she has been taken and the man has easy daily access to the bedroom, this dance does not continue. So women find it outside the home in stories or movies to feed their imagination with a fantasy world.

This is another reason why women can be just as tempted as men in having an affair. They want to feel loved and ravaged with all their body sensations on fire. To complicate the matter, once the reptile brain has been satisfied, a woman shifts to the higher brain functions needing more emotional connection for the long-term relationship. She cannot survive solely on the reptile urgings. You cannot raise a family by allowing these urges to dominate and dictate otherwise other problems arise.

A young child might not cope with the shocking visions of their parent's bodies smashing, groaning and screaming as they once did on the kitchen table or on top of the sink. The child becomes fearful that the father is hurting the mother and the child thinks his life could be threatened too. This is potentially a great recipe for psychological damage. So a female will generally become mindful of the child's mental and emotional development and resort to keeping her sexual needs and fantasies hidden—hidden for years and years.

Fear of Pregnancy STOPS SEX!

The biggest fear a woman carries with her with every sexual act is the fear of an unplanned pregnancy. This event can change her whole life immeasurably and irrevocably. Men, and even some women, might think the idea of abortion is an easy solution, but I have never seen much evidence of this when women speak up about their true feelings. It's instinctual when a woman conceives, and life even in its simplest form, has begun within her, the BODY wants to take that process to full term. It's no different from a man holding back his sperm release just before it's about to release. Will that ever happen? Rarely! They might pull out and then release, but still they let it go. This is the power and the mind of the BODY'S need to continue the survival of the species and not necessarily listen to the emotional, mental needs of the person. There is no guarantee that once a woman becomes pregnant that some mighty force of thinking within her does not override common sense, current lifestyle plans and future goals. All that can be gone in an instant, once the creation process takes place within the body.

So when it comes to sex, there is always a small possibility to become pregnant especially during the most exciting time of ovulation, even when taking precautions. There are plenty of stories of pregnancy happening even with contraception. I say exciting time of ovulation, because this is the natural time of the month when the female's body is programmed and ready to become pregnant, so it's obvious she wants more sex then. Her BODY wants to get pregnant. This is her cycle, the same style of cycle that links us to the animal world. If we have a pet that goes into heat, we lock them up when it's their cycle if we don't want them to become pregnant. If we don't, the female will prowl the streets displaying her needs alerting all the males in the area. Cows will bellow: Come get me.

This is just another reason why men might not get to play nearly as much as they would like to. Their female partner is filled with a secret anxiety and wants to avoid the decision of having another baby or feeling forced to decide on an abortion. How sad it is for a woman, when it comes to the most exciting part of the month when she is most likely to enjoy knees-to-the-ears, rip-roaring sex, that a little voice inside her says, "Careful, this could be the time when it all goes wrong." So she holds back, possibly avoids sex altogether, if she is that intuitively in touch with her own cycle. What can be done? *Double, triple contraception coverage?* That's not appealing, but worth thinking about.

There are extremes to prevent pregnancy. For example, a woman can have a hysterectomy but then she becomes menopausal and ferocious and no man or woman really wants that too early in the relationship. So what will it take for a woman to not worry about an unplanned pregnancy? A woman can have her tubes tied, a man can have a vasectomy, and still after all that men might want to use a condom. Talk together about this to make sure this is not just one more issue getting in the way of enjoying deep loving relations.

Possible Solution? Sex during Menstruation. There is another way to have sex in the time of month that is considered quite safe—during menstruation. Women often feel quite horny at this time. There might not be a rhyme or reason behind it, but those amorous feelings do arise, perhaps because she is safe from creating babies. Now it is not common to hear of people having sex during this time, as it's not something they will admit to freely, but it can and does happen. It also can be enjoyable, especially if the couple showers together, as this eliminates a sense of mess and self-consciousness on the woman's part and visually, might be just too much for the male to take in. Of course, sex will be far more enjoyable if the woman doesn't have a heavy flow. On a physical level, menstrual cramps can be greatly relieved if the female experiences an orgasm during this time.

The other really positive psychological gain a woman can get from making love during this time is the overwhelming feeling that she is being loved and accepted for every part of being a woman—even the part that she might feel appalled by on a monthly basis.

CAUTION: Having sex during menses is not risk free, as there is higher risk of infection and a higher sexually transmitted diseases (STD) rate, due to the cervix being slightly open. Pregnancy could still happen.

It is not easy for me to speak about this, because I know there are women who feel so relieved each month knowing there is a break from the constant demands of sex from their partners. By sharing this knowledge, I might be taking away the one time of peace she looks forward to each month. However, there are also many women who would love to experience stress-free sex without the fears of getting pregnant. So, I have had to think deeply before speaking about this and sharing my story.

My first real sexual relationship was with a man I ended up living with for four years. He was experienced in the art of love-making. He made me feel precious, loved, revered and above all respected, as he slowly introduced me to the many joys of my own body. His patience was astounding with my blossoming sexuality. I was an open book for him and he treated me with respect. He seemed to take great pleasure and pride in himself to open this new world to me. One day when I was menstruating, we began to kiss and touch but before we went any further, I told him it was not possible today.

Instead of being put off by this, he gently and lovingly led me to the shower. As he kissed me and took off my clothes, he whispered a reassurance that it was completely possible to make love when menstruating, if you find a way to clean up as you go. I can only say it was one of the most beautiful experiences I have had in my sexual life because not only did I feel completely accepted and loved as a woman, but it somehow was exotically sensuous and my body sensations all seemed heightened.

I will say that it took quite a bit of convincing. He, who had the gift of words, reassured me that other women did this and enjoyed the whole experience. Fortunately, I am not a heavy bleeder so I tentatively decided to explore this new experience. How did he know that many other women enjoyed this, you might ask? Well, he ended up being a pathological player before, during and, I would suspect, after our relationship. Regardless of the reasons for breaking up, I am grateful for his teaching and guidance in these matters. He provided a fantastic foundation and helped me feel comfortable within my own sexuality.

SPECIAL NOTE: Some women experience period-like bleedings twice a month. Once is the normal menstrual time of the uterus clearing out the old lining to make way for the new lining. The other time is OVULATION TIME, baby-making time. If you are a woman, this happens to, then make sure you know exactly where you are in your cycle, because if you are not on any form of contraception, you should not risk getting pregnant.

Body Weight

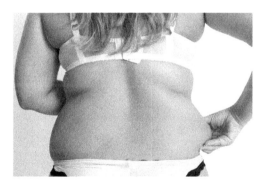

How the woman perceives her body and what she THINKS it looks like from a man's eyes can drastically affect how comfortable she is with sex. Everything changes in a woman's body after a baby—stretch marks, floppy skin, drastic weight gain or perceived weight gain and interior and exterior vaginal changes can all play havoc with the mind of the woman. Depending on her initial level of self-confidence and ease in the bedroom, a woman might have a varying degree of internal anxiety dialogue.

Now, when you read these possible thoughts of a woman you will immediately think that this dialogue of paranoia is only for women who are grossly overweight or suffering obesity. In fact, these are also thoughts that many women within minimal weight gain will also think and especially after a baby is born, as the tone of the abdomen might not have tightened up as quick as she would like.

A Women's Thoughts Are Her Greatest Enemy

These thoughts include the following:

Floppy Stomach—"I avoid taking the top position because my floppy stomach will jiggle in front of his eyes and he will be turned off."

Stretch Marks—"I hope he does not look at my ugly stretch marks," followed by subtly trying to cover them with her hands if he is exploring her body.

Vagina—"Oh, no, please don't look down there. It doesn't look pretty anymore."

Nipples—Trying to redirect the nipple nibbling to other areas because the nipples are no longer sensitive and the act is annoying or hurts. Thinking "I hope I didn't hurt him by pushing him away." Also, the breasts might have lost a lot of their fullness after children, as babies seem to suck the fat tissue from them, drastically changing their form. This is more evident after multiple children, but saggy breasts can also be a problem.

Doggy Style—"Can he feel all the flubber swinging in the breeze? Oh, no, he just grabbed a handful of flab."

Man on Top—"I'm not sure how long I will be able to breathe before I have to push him off," as the man lovingly hammers away on top of the woman. The fat of her stomach is pushing with great force on the diaphragm and essentially the woman feels as if she is going to suffocate. This makes it hard to allow for sufficient relaxation to occur for orgasm.

All these thoughts can affect the woman as she lies alongside her partner and the anxiety begins to rise. As each anxious thought forms within the mind, the more stressed and uncomfortable she becomes, eventually causing her vaginal moisture to suddenly dry up, or a general stiffness in her otherwise fluidic lovemaking. These are sure signs that some kind of disconnect has occurred within the female mind and could mean that she perhaps needs to talk about her phobias.

Negotiate new ways to navigate around her body until her confidence builds up once again. Perhaps, even though she will feel humiliated to enter conversation about this openly, it will help her get those thoughts and feelings out on the table. You can reassure her how you feel about her and how attractive she is in your eyes. New body positions can be negotiated to perhaps help body discomfort. They did not create the Karma Sutra thousands of years ago for no reason. *Explore your body, explore your partner.*

Body Odor and Sexual Fluids

Women become paranoid with their own vaginal smell. If they detect their own strong odor, they will tend to try to avoid sexual activity at that time. Odor can occur for a variety of reasons. At different times of the month as the cycle of menstruation is looming, hormonal releases change the odor. Many men can detect those changes and some, after being in a relationship for a long time, will know a woman's cycle according to those changes.

Some food choices will change the vaginal odor. Garlic can change the whole body aroma and often release a sour pungent smell. This is great on food but not always on the body. Digestive disturbances can be a formidable cause of vaginal odor. When the digestive system is not functioning as it should, gases and toxins create chemical changes in the mucosa of the body. The vagina is a moist environment made up of mucous membranes, so it is a primary area where the chemical changes occur.

Vaginal changes can also be due to a condition referred to as **Bacterial Vaginitis**. This is a situation where an overgrowth of one or more bacteria upset the natural balance of the vagina resulting in an inflammation process. Any woman can experience the condition but it's more prevalent during a ladies reproductive years. It would appear certain sexual activities might increase the likelihood of onset. Symptoms can be quite uncomfortable and be experienced as insane itching, discharge and pain. Tampons, condoms, neglected diaphragms, irritating douches and deodorant sprays could place you at higher risk.

The most common types of vaginitis are:

- **Candida Albicans** is regarded by natural therapists as a friendly fungal bacteria in the intestinal tract but when the bacteria becomes overgrown it causes many imbalances and the bacteria can then find its way to the vagina causing labia swelling and white discharge. It is also responsible for abdominal bloating and discomfort.
- **Trichomoniasis**, is caused by a sexually transmitted parasite resulting in a foul discharge and odor. Can be worse in pregnancy.

- **Vaginal atrophy (atrophic vaginitis),** which results from reduced estrogen levels during menopause.
- **Bacterial Vaginosis** is a non-specific vaginitis associated with positive cultures of Garnerella Vaginalis causing fishy odours.

Ladies, there are ways to remedy most of these embarrassing situations so you can continue having relaxed and enjoyable sexual interactions. Medical help is available, but there are many options within the natural alternative fields of therapy to help. Visit a local Naturopath and he or she will guide you in the right direction so you can once again enjoy a stress-free sex life.

Sperm Etiquette

There is an unspoken etiquette about what should be done with sperm after lovemaking sessions. With most sexual encounters with a male orgasm, seminal fluid follows. Now this fluid might remain in the condom or within the woman's vagina, but often some leaks out. So everyone needs to know it's not like the movies when the couple lovingly lays cradled in each other's arms without a care in the world. There is usually a cold wet patch somewhere underneath that one of you will roll onto and one of you might heartily be avoiding by rolling the other secretly onto that patch because you don't want to sleep in it. This can give rise to amusement with each other and other times resentment. So for this reason I have added this next section on sperm etiquette.

Women don't have to worry about leaving behind wet patches unless they too ejaculate (some women do express fluid when they have an orgasm). Men, on the other hand, can often leave fluid around that has not remained within the walls of the vagina or has been purposefully deposited somewhere else. Men sometimes feel a little awkward about where their sperm has gone (only after the fact) in relation to what kind of sexual play is at hand. This could be something they have fantasized or are a little horrified about. So for mutual respect, it's really important for the man to take some responsibility toward his own fluid in way of cleaning up, but the woman should also be gentle, kind and helpful toward this cleanup process. Negative comments at this time could really injure the man's ego because of his perception of rejection or criticism of his internal creation.

Everyone is different, but within an established relationship, many of you have already discovered some common sense about this process. It is an important thing to be open for discussion, because there are some parts of the lovemaking sexual act that might literally gross your partner out, but he or she has never spoken about it. Each time if the same issue arises, eventually avoidance becomes the outcome. Some women are more experimental than others are. You need to know who is in your playground, how they are feeling about any one session and what personal lines are drawn about how you play with each other. If she feels intimate and cuddly needing reassurance, but the man chooses to re-enacts his deepest fantasies at that time, then it really is a recipe for disaster. Sensitivity is the key.

SO...

Ejaculating and then rubbing it proudly all over her, laying down on top of her after releasing on her body, then squishing it all about might not be well received, nor will having the ejaculate directed at her hair or eyes. Filled condoms that are carelessly spilled everywhere, coming all over her face without prior consent, not warning her that you are about to ejaculate in her mouth, forcing her mouth to stay wrapped around your shaft by holding her head are NOT considered showing respect for your partner. There are many other scenarios possible but I think you get the picture. You need to have a mutual agreement about what feels safe and comfortable for the other.

{ 4 }

Hints to Understand Your Man

Power of the Hand Job

"I am so worked up, I can't think straight."
"It's been months since we last made love."

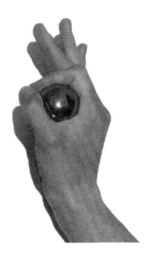

Did I just say hand job? Shock! Horror!

I know, as a woman, I can barely spit those words out, but someone has to be the men's spokesperson and it's better to come from a woman than a man, otherwise he will be accused of self-interest. So ladies, the men have a story too—if the man is stressed, sex is the answer. If he is carrying obvious stress then the kindest thing a woman can do is give him a hand in releasing the male pressure. If you can't do the full sexual intimate contact because you feel as if it's an invasion of your private space, then let him lie there and give him a hand or head job. When you hear him sleeping, be happy that you have skills that give him a great and understanding sleeping pill. He will respond in many open communicative ways in the days that follow. Better still, whenever possible, join him in the shower. Lather each other's body with soap. Care for one another. This is a lovely way to explore your partner's body in a caring and respectful manner. It is also the language of love for a woman, as touching and stroking with the silken effects of the soap is very sensuous. In this way women can still experience immense enjoyment even when not pursuing personal fulfillment via orgasm. Dare I say that a man could also demonstrate the same care for a woman without him pursuing his own orgasm. In this way you will show your partner how much you care and are not acting with self-interest.

For those men who have a real aversion to a hand job then there might be an underlying psychological issue that needs investigation and support.

Painful Blue-Ball Syndrome

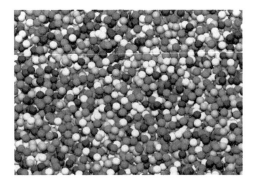

There is a valid physical reason behind encouraging a partner to help take pressure off the male's genitals. There is a condition commonly known as blue balls. Men can suffer this if they have not had sex for a long time or if they have anticipated that foreplay would result in orgasm and for some reason this possibility is interrupted. Unreleased sperm can cause the testicles to swell to double their size and the extra blood in the immediate area causes the scrotum to appear blue. Men can feel extreme pain in the local area of the scrotum and also penetrating throughout the abdominal region. This pain can cause aggression and short temperedness. It is this condition that can also add to the man needing to masturbate for release if he is not sexually active enough.

Women also can experience blue ovaries. Now I can't say that the ovaries swell up to double the size but I can say that when a women is excited through extensive foreplay and sexual activity does not result in orgasm, she can experience incredible pain ripping through her lower abdomen, leaving her with a lack of sexual relief. This might not happen to all women but through my own experience as a young virgin enjoying heavy petting I would go to my mother with these pains. She explained this was the result and effect of heavy kissing and told me to stop what I was doing, as it was not good for me but especially unfair to the young man. Embarrassed, I decided to make a mental note and sure enough each time we began kissing without an end I would experience pain.

This same situation arose at times in married life when children interrupted those special intimate times. Pains would arise but immediately subside when followed through with orgasm or sometimes with deep penetration without orgasm. I have since learned through talking to other women that this is more common than realized or talked about, often the discomfort was explained away as something completely different.

Falling to Sleep after Sex

Testicles are a Sperm Factory! There are 20–40 million microscopic sperm created per milliliter within an ejaculate. That's enough sperm to begin populating a planet in one ejaculation! Each sperm is packed full of nutrients extracted from the male body's daily energy requirements. Hormones, minerals, vitamins and amino acids siphoned from the main system are all pumped into the testicles in order to create new life. It stands to reason that men are completely, biologically exhausted after releasing their life-giving sperm. They state that no matter how hard they try to remain attentive after sex they still become overwhelmed by fatigue.

Men report their bodies feel tired, they long for sleep, ears buzz, eyes are heavy, they are thirsty and their limbs feel stiff and weak. After ejaculating, he will only enjoy brief moments of pleasurable sensations before becoming completely overwhelmed by long hours of exhaustion. For days after, a man's mental clarity and body energy will be dulled. This is why athletes are encouraged to not have sex prior to events. Many creative artists also have recognized the link between sex and lessened creative mind power.

Why Do Women Stroke and Not Grope?

Women tend to touch the man the way they like to be touched—by stroking, gently, softly, alluring. Women tend to have all these heightened senses in the fingertips that course through her body with pleasure signals. Her body parts like to be stroked like a delicate flower, so she strokes when she is feeling happy and it signals to the man her openness and happiness. However, she can linger and stroke for hours on end, never taking this gentle stimulation any further. It's her greatest loving touch. It borders on sacredness from within and she is gifting that to a man. If a man wants to be part of this woman's gift, he needs to return the favor with stroking. *Caution: Testicles are sensitive, so allow the man show you how to approach.*

Ladies, if you want to cuddle when you sleep or sit on the couch being held, then you have to keep your stroking fingers at bay, otherwise this will tell the man that he can begin his first amorous male moves on you. It's his permission slip. If you want his mind to remain stable and not begin definite sexual advances, then you must act more like a man—sitting uncommitted on the couch or laying in bed. No tenderness on its own, otherwise you invite the bedroom song.

Groping Is a Man's Touch of Love

A man loves to get right to the business. He shows love by grabbing what he wants. This is an alpha male behavior and can become exciting and intoxicating in the early days of a relationship, and even at times in a mature relationship, but not every time he comes near your body. Women will often shy away from too much heavy-handed, grabbing and grasping, but the man is different.

He wants you to get down to business, demanding what you want from him because he is eager to gift you with his style of loving and deposit. He wants you to grab, squeeze and pull because he has the greatest gift to give—potential life. He wants you to hunger for it as he hungers to give it. So women, sometimes you have to step up to the mark to add that extra excitement in the relationship and give him the thrill of his life.

Watch your partner's body language and look for any negative reactions around your use of stroking. For some men, it can be, quite frankly, annoying.

Don't Criticize Sexual Clumsiness

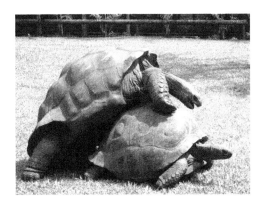

There might be times, especially at the onset of a new relationship, where the man might appear clumsy or does not handle your body well. This might be due to a complete lack of experience, or no one has gently guided him to the workings of the female body. It is my hope that after reading this book that both sexes might actually navigate the sexual arena of their lives with more knowledge and understanding.

If you dearly love the man and really want the relationship to last the distance, you will need to help him. Show him and explain how your body works without using critical words or ridiculing him. He is much more sensitive than you realize. He might not be able to hold back his excitement in the beginning, but if you find he can't hold it back once you are an established couple then more work is needed. He needs to learn how to keep his excited thoughts in check by thinking of something else. Thankfully, now at a touch of the button with the Internet so much help is available for men and women in this department. It is a time like this when you might want to initiate the changes.

Performance terror in new relationships might be a factor in what appears as sexual clumsiness but is quite different. The man might not be able to harden up sufficiently for a sexual encounter. Men can become insanely nervous and uptight about how they will measure up. Sometimes the more they think about it, the worse they become. Be patient and take your time. If there is evidence from the past that something is mentally or emotionally bothering the man, and he will not talk about it with you, then he might need outside professional support by way of a counseling or medical appointment.

To Initiate or Not

This is a tricky subject and where men can get confusing. Many men love a woman to initiate intimacy, as it takes the pressure off possible rejection. It's a huge relief to know there will be positive action to the night. Married men in particular need definite positive cues, because by the time many years have passed in the relationship they are as confused as hell and often just give up trying. There is only so much rejection a man can take.

Having said that, I have met many women who have spoken about their attempts to initiate intimacy, and it has turned the man completely off his game. This has caused the woman to deal with her insecurities and then never know if she should ever try again. Not only did the woman initiate sex but she dared to climb on top of the man, only to discover a limp, disastrous end. Horrified and confused, she assumed she has revolted the man. That never ends well. They both end up in therapy.

Generally speaking, men like to be the hunter, the aggressor and he TAKES his woman. "UGH!" It fills him with alpha male importance and dominance. He feels in control and loves to think that every act he attempts on the women is going to thrill her to the core and she will be bucking, weaving and heaving with delightful convulsions when he gives it to her. That is his joy and the language he was built for.

Sometimes when a man is known to respond to a women's invitation with definite rejection, it can usually be traced to memories in his earlier life. He might need some counseling or psychological support, unless the woman understands his need to be the dominant male and is happy to let him take over and remain in control. A woman can try a less aggressive approach to start the foreplay by sending subtle stroking messages to help him be aware of the invitation. This will usually allow him to take over and think it was his idea. **BEWARE:** Don't stroke, if you don't want a poke.

Temptations—Men and the Wandering Eye

So I've talked about boring predictability and the female emotional needs but incessant rejections and avoidance tactics can also bore men. Nagging that never seems to abate aggravate their boredom level. A woman who is constantly dissatisfied with her life and offers constant critical abuse, negativity and sexual rejection, can cause a man to feel demoralized and unloved. This places him in a state of potential wandering thoughts and eyes. No human wants to walk the planet feeling as if he or she is the plague. Sooner or later, a man will want to feel whole, loved, appreciated, accepted and sexually attractive. So a time might come when the man can no longer maintain his loyalty in the marital bed, no matter how hard he tries or how long he has withheld. Most men do not want to deliberately risk their partnership, children's security or financial freedom, but their anatomy pushes them to override their reason, in moments of weakness. Battered emotional states can also propel them to look for understanding, emotional and physical, elsewhere.

Women need to find within themselves a generosity of spirit to help prevent the possible wandering thoughts and keep the man fully focused at home.

Men DO Like to Be Listened To

Through many years of living with men in our life, we might come to faultily assume that men don't actually want to talk or express themselves in emotional ways. It is quite the opposite. If men did not want to be heard, listened to or express their innermost thoughts and feelings, even as they age, why is it that they share so deeply with a new woman when having an affair or starting a new relationship? This is often to the point that they become gushingly romantic! The cynic would say just to get to the bedroom, but really, in those early parts of relationship building and sharing, men open up and share deeply personal things, sometimes even shocking themselves.

The female in the early stages of a relationship also loves openly and does not go into habitual negative behavior by interlacing her listening with comments of negativity, criticism, blame, neediness, guilt or call him up on his male responsibilities. This makes a perfect safe, space for men to feel heard and valued. When a man opens up and listens without expectation or comment, his deepest emotional self comes forward and it's easy for him to believe he is in love as he spills his insides out. Men DO need to be heard and valued! Sadly it is often the environment of long-term relationships, with a whole host of convoluted ingredients, that makes it so hard for each partner to feel safe to open up honestly and fully. Personal feelings, hurts, perceptions and FEARS seep into relating to the partner, potentially destroying what was once a beautiful powerful thread of communication that was the glue to join the relationship in the first instance. New relationships and affairs begin with open communication, but it does not take long for men to assume the silent position that is so familiar for them when hints of criticism, nagging or neediness enter the conversations.

Men's Confusion about Women Dressing Up

During all the years I've been counseling, I've had many men express their frustration, insecurities and sometimes anger about their partner dressing up extensively to go out. It's often a man's perception that women dress up to attract other men. They become agitated, because for years they've been missing out on sex, not searching for it elsewhere and forever loyal, only to see their partner dress up and parade out of the home. To a man's view, the woman is advertising herself for a potential sexual encounter. It can drive him nuts. Of course, I've met men who are the opposite—they love to show off what they have at home and can actually encourage or pressure the woman to present in a certain way, sometimes to the detriment of the relationship. Women are often worse than men in this respect, frequently dictating to the man about how to dress and placing them outside their comfort zone, making the man feel agitated and confused.

I'll let you in on a secret that every woman doesn't really realize. Many women dress for other women. Not in a homosexual way, but to actually compete with one another. Women are more interested to see how many men's heads turn to them instead of the other women in the group, down the street or at events. The increase of male attention lifts their low self-esteem. They feel connected to the game of life, but never in their wildest dreams are they thinking to take action if a man was to look or to offer his sexual services to her. Most women would be horrified to think their dressing up is interpreted in this way.

For those women who have been accused, they become mortally wounded and angry that a partner could even think that of them. Women use cloths of color and texture to express their inner being and how they feel. Oftentimes it's a mask to cover feelings of inner conflict, self-doubt and self-loathing. They use clothes and makeup to turn heads and boost self-esteem. They'll equally feel like crap quite quickly if someone else looks fabulous and has all heads turning. They like heads turning to appreciate them, and it's not about wanting to have sex.

It's these thoughts, actions and insecurities that have women always asking their partner if they look good in the clothes they are wearing. It's to feel reassured and good that their partner finds them pleasing and he'll be proud to walk with them in public. Women get agitated when a man says he likes everything. In fact, he would probably rather see her naked and available for sex before they go out, so he can take her and own her without sharing her with men doing the eye feast. He needs reassurance that she is not wanting to look great and saving herself for other men's attention.

Of course, there is always the deep-seated element of a woman wanting proof she is still attractive to the opposite sex, but her thoughts are not daily, hourly, consumed by this or the sexual act. Her mind's attention on this is subtle and hidden, embedded in the animal psyche. By now, she's moved on from that being her motivating factor.

Men, you need to understand this because you have a huge influence toward making or breaking a woman's belief in herself. If a woman is complimented and reassured that you find her really attractive whether she is dressed up, wearing bags, or naked, then there is a high chance for sexual action. No matter her shape or weight, if you can find the love language for the woman, she will blossom and your needs will be met more often.

Ladies—Most Men Don't Like Makeup

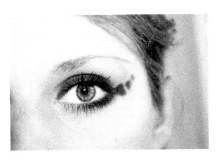

Throughout the years of my personal dating, subsequent marriage and becoming a mother of teenage boys, I get the same message. This is backed up by hundreds of men in the clinic. Most men don't like makeup. They don't like the taste or the smell. They don't like it on their clothes. They also think it looks ridiculous. Many men really enjoy the simple and practical beauty of a naked face and skin. They like to experience the image of before and after of dating and mating to be the same. In their minds, makeup says the woman is open for sexual business. Paradoxically though, the women who are extensively masked and cannot go out of the house without having their face covered are often covering many insecurities and low self-worth, which makes them much less emotionally available and more likely to reject.

Teenage boys complain about this in their dating. Heavily made-up girls are intimidating to them due to the frequency of rejection, even though she is dressed and made up to gain maximum attention, or so he thinks. They don't realize the girls dress to cover inadequacies of mental and emotional processing and to compete with other girls. Those girls who have no need to join the peer group are usually, but not always, more stable with personal confidence and much more likely to accept the attention. When more men and boys pursue the attentions of the natural girls and not fixate on cleavage and miniskirts then societal attitudes might eventually change. Women will feel freer to be themselves, trust-ing their natural attractiveness.

Ladies, dress the way you feel most comfortable. Be aware of your actions and the possible need to hide how you really feel or not. Decide what makes you personally feel good, but don't compete with other women. That is only fraught with personal danger of undermining your inner balance. Know that men love the natural look of you. His eyes might gaze on others, but he'll always feel consumed with love at home when you do your best to be available for him to express his form of loving.

If all your childhood role models wore makeup, then you might have been conditioned that this is what women must do to be a real woman. It might be time to reexamine those conditionings.

Men Are Not Mind Readers—Ask or Demonstrate

What is it with women that they expect the man to know what they are thinking? She hints toward an idea rather than asking for what she wants done. In the bedroom, you have to begin showing him how to touch you. I know you stroke his body, but he does not interpret that as you wanting him to stroke your whole body or vaginal regions in the same way. Remember, men are visual. Grab his hand and show him. The first couple of times he might not get the idea right in his head, because by him looking at you touching yourself and realizing that he gets to see you do that, well, he won't be able to hold back for long.

Sadly, a woman is actually turned off by having to be so bla-tant as to show the man what he should, in her view, instinctively know. It takes the power and mystery away from the moment. It's too physical, too practical. Women hate practical, especially in the bedroom. They want to stay in a swooning altered state engaging the heightened senses of the right brain where ecstasy, love and passion exist.

What about the home front? We expect our partners to know exactly what we want help with and we expect that they will just see what is to be done and do it. Why do they need to be constantly directed like a child? Well, men can only do one thing at a time, because they are left-brain dominant and sequential in their life approach. This frustrates the hell out of women, as they feel like they have another child in their midst. If you women can learn to be honest and just speak up about what you need, men will mostly be happy to help and assist, especially if they get a little bonus bit of loving from you from time to time rather than receiving a ranting, raging maelstrom of words for their efforts. They also need encouragement, otherwise they will shrink.

Men Love Deeply

Kindness and gentle words go a long way. Men essentially are really soft inside. They love deeply—much more than women give them credit for. Every waking hour, when they are not thinking about sex, they are thinking about how they can make their family life better, fulfill their partner's expectations of life they will do whatever it takes to make that dream a reality. Many men drive themselves to the wall through overwork just to give the woman what he thinks she wants. What he thinks she wants is the big house, better clothes, dance classes for the kids and holidays because she mentions them a lot.

What women really want is to be understood, nurtured, emotionally supported and someone to share the huge role of parenting. They also want to be seen as an individual with as many needs to discover who she is as a man does. She might like the material things, but if there is no emotional support in the home, she can easily walk away from it all. When women walk out of the relationship, this surprises men and then angers them. They have invested huge amounts of time and energy into a working life, thinking it is all worthwhile even if he is getting less sexual reward than he would like. Stunned he realizes just how much of his personal dreams have been eaten up while he has been concentrating on the comforts and needs of his partner and family. Left to his own devices he would have made different decisions. A man's dream does not usually involve sitting in an office chair away from sunlight for 40–50 years of his life. He does it for his family and for his retirement, when he looks forward to having his partner to himself again. No kids, no distractions. They want to live in the castle they spent a lifetime building.

Male Suppression—Nagging Negative Partners

Where does the need to nag come from? Why is there the need to actively jump on any ideas a man has by immediately voiding it with comments? Why do women just say NO to an idea or desired action before thinking about it? I ask you these questions because I pondered on them heavily myself and realized the reason I believe why women are quick to jump or comment on a man's ideas is because the woman believes he is just talking like women do on random comments. He's just throwing an idea into the mix without really having any need for it to go further than discussion.

We might not always stop to think that the man might have actually mentioned something important to him and his personal needs as an individual on the planet. Instead, we quickly assume and often tear them apart by negative comments. It's human nature, but if this happens too much in a relationship then the man (and indeed it happens a lot to women) becomes suppressed and an inner volcano of emotions begins festering under the surface.

So it's really important as women that we come to know that many men spend much of their married lives trying to keep their partners happy and operating in a balanced way. Before they ever dare to mention their ideas, thoughts or feelings, many men ponder and weigh their needs to express an opinion long before a women ever knows about it. When the man finally speaks up, it is usually tentative, hoping he will be listened to and the subject will be given due consideration by his partner.

With this entire internal dialogue of plans and opinions going on, men can react strongly to the nagging intensity and negative tirades that might fall out of the lips of partners. They will resist, become passively noncompliant, sad and submissive or become verbal as they make a stand for their needs.

Now, ladies, I know we can feel exactly the same way but we KNOW we feel like this, however, we don't often stop to think that a man, who usually puts his family first, might also have hidden dreams and needs for new challenges, experiences, life goals, adventures or mental stimulation. They do, but mostly they keep their thoughts private and hidden to the point that they do not even know how to express those needs. When they actually speak up or mention their idea or needs, it's imperative that our ears of intuition prick up and take note because those needs, if ignored or overlooked, can sometimes be make-or-break moments of the relationship.

Who Lives in This House Anyway?

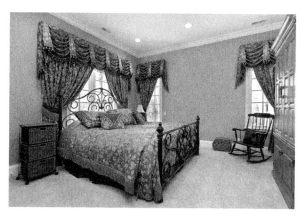

Another form of accidental suppression that can happen to either a man or woman are the choices of décor, renovations or amount of space in which a person is allowed to express their own personal individual essence of oneself in the home.

In counseling, when women come in feeling unheard, not valued, respected or listened to, or they feel threatened with the man spending more time away from the home, it alerts me to certain potential issues. They might mention he is spending more time with friends, run away to other activities or shut down and become more distant. When this happens, I usually ask one question:

What does your bedroom look like? Who designed the décor? Is there anything in the bedroom that represents the man's interests or nature, especially his nature and interests before you came into his life?

I am usually faced with blank, stunned looks but then I watch their mind visualize all the frilly curtains, ornaments, color schemes, perfumes, shoes, overfilled closets spilling into the man's side. They might even see that every shelf in the bathroom area is filled with girl items, with only a small section put aside for a razor and maybe, if they are lucky, some pills for a hangover. The pills also might be on the girl side for menstrual cramps. Then when he needs them, he has to go digging among tampons, pungent perfumes, nail polish and all manner of non-identifiable objects.

As the internal mental process unfolds, a light of understanding emanates from their eyes. I follow it up with, "So now you tell me, WHO is listening to whom and valuing the other person's need to express oneself? Who in this scenario might be feeling suppressed? Who was the first person to stop listening?

These questions can be confronting and are genuinely asked in a gentle non-judging manner, holding the space so the person might be able to view herself and her actions with a balanced mind. For all relationships to unfold in a loving, accepting way, both parties have to take responsibility for their own actions. Now I know I have fixated on women being the interior decorator, as this is the usual issue that is raised by men coming in for support. Having said that, I apologize to all those women who have also felt the same style of suppression in their homes.

What Men Tell Me. Men often come in not knowing why they feel depressed for no real reason and have lost their drive to improve their lives or make more effort in their relationships. The first thing they might mention is the onslaught of criticism and nagging, causing them to feel they can't do anything right. They might also talk about their sex life becoming nonexistent and this hurts and confuses them. On deeper exploration, they emotionally burst out, that it's been like this since they first moved in with their partner and the whole house was transformed before their eyes.

Every article, picture, hobby that reflected his personality was abolished to the spare room or a private hideaway or shed. He suddenly found himself in a woman's world of frilly cushions, excessive pillows on the bed, color schemes changing to girl tastes and he could no longer put his hands on the razor that always sat on the counter so it was easy to find. In the spare room all his hobby items that he could see and pick up on the run, now were hidden among a clutter of other less important hobby items, tools tossed aside, damaged university furniture filled with hilarious memories of boys being boys. Effectively HE has been eradicated as his new love moves in.

This female takeover might be outwardly accepted, as the practical solution in the sharing of space and his quiet compliance is an attempt to shows his love of the incoming resident, but secretly the man often feels that from the outset, his old self has been criticized and rejected. Now, years later, and the same scenarios are recreating, whittling down his reserves and personality expression. He finds himself sick, despondent, with no drive and often a lagging sexual drive as he has felt progressively neutered as a man. He has morphed into a man–woman, internally tortured.

This story keeps repeating itself during the life of the partnership, unless the couple can find a safe space to bring up these issues and have their mutual needs met. This is easier said than done. Women have a huge amount of advertising pitted against them, and they are susceptible to popular reactions among peers. These external driving factors make it hard for them to listen and value the man. An unsaid compromise usually unfolds. The shed or fishing shack is the man's domain. OR is it?

Here comes the new battlefront. Home renovation shows that encourage the takeover of a man's beloved shed have a lot to answer for. Now his only sanctum, the private space away from the home filled with his nostalgic memories and man pheromones of caveman proportions is suddenly invaded. Fond memories whisked away by sweet-smelling cleaning agents emanating from the fecal-encrusted toilet bowl. Fancy reflective outdoor kitchens replace the ramshackle bar made from the top of a surfboard, and the old fridge (posing as a dartboard) has gone to the dump.

Friends no longer gravitate to hang out in the renovated shed, as the women and children do their silent takeover into the once man-only domain. Nagging about who cleans the toilet and shed becomes commonplace, where once the man was left to his own mysterious man cave activities. High-pitched tones of a female voice invade like a serpent ready to strike.

The Hunter Feels Hunted

Society has slowly been hunting the man down and neutering him. Every man domain is becoming feminized and sanitized. It all started with the public bars. In earlier generations, not that long ago, the public bar was for MEN ONLY. This was a place that was not deemed appropriate for fine, upstanding, genteel ladies to go. They were allocated a separate area for ladies called the lounge area.

The public bar was a place where men could express themselves openly and do business. They could swear without offending, release internal gas and make jokes, let out huge beer-filled burps, slug another beer down the hatch and make unsavory, lewd remarks to the cleavage-showing barmaid in a pathetic attempt to flirt. All the while forgetting they were sporting an overly large beer-barrel stomach, long time removed from their rippling abs of yesteryear.

Men were happy and content to be in a place where they could speak without getting in trouble and say the most profound things about an overly exaggerated work event among guffaws of laughter amidst contributions of further ridiculous and random comments. All of this was expressed among a brotherhood of men who understood and did not criticize them. A place they felt accepted and their manhood celebrated.

This might be all good for their happy brain chemical production, perhaps not so good for their wallet, home finances or distressed wives.

Having spent many years in my 20s as a bartender as I traveled and then settled into bar work in a regular Australian town, I witnessed many of these things. I came to realize how important it was for men to have this space. It was also what I would consider my first step into the world of counseling and listening and I would thoroughly recommend this type of work to anyone thinking of moving into a career of counseling or men's support.

My generation came after many public bars were invaded by women, as it became more acceptable for women to join the men. However, I saw and felt attitudes and behavior change, especially among the older gentlemen, when a woman entered the bar. Stories normally interlaced with colorful swear words would be shut off with apologies if the female stumbled on the last lewd comments. All conversations were adjusted to be suitable for a lady to listen to and join in. Even as a bartender, the men would hush their guttural words if I was passing by or serving that area of the bar. Other times they felt comfortable enough to reveal a fair measure of their truest selves or when their lips loosened from alcohol lubrication. Back then, many men did not have the income for the luxury of a private space or shed. The public bar was their shed.

Women descending into the men's bar area had men changing their meeting habits. The men turned to men-only fishing and hunting trips, and as income rose, they purchased fishing shanty shacks and backyard sheds. Now these are becoming extinct, as women lace up their humble living quarters and demand major renovations. Once again this eradicates his personality imprint and expression of being. Where to next?

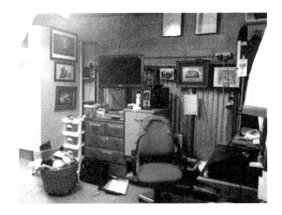

Public Created Men Sheds—How sad that now, due to such a lack of understanding and downsizing for old age, the man loses his space and the place where his friends could find him. Pubs are too expensive to drink in and have often morphed into glitzy upmarket establishments to keep up with the ever-changing demands of the new younger clientele. All over the world, a new culture has emerged. Public men spaces are being created for general use. This is in answer to a man's desperate need to belong to a tribe he understands and feels accepted in. If, as a society, we have to create such places, surely it is showing us that somewhere the lack of understanding among the sexes has gone desperately wrong and needs review.

Women, if you want your partner to really flourish like you want to flourish, then be more gentle and understanding of the man's needs. This will go a long way toward him softening to you and perhaps deeper communication and emotional connection can be reinvigorated. You never know when more sexual attention and lovingness might follow. I sincerely hope this explains a lot of changing emotions and possible tensions that might arise in the relationship you cherish and do not want to lose.

{ 5 }
Sexual Extras

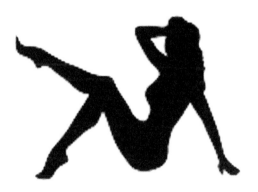

Highly Sexed Women Exist

Don't get me wrong with all this negative talk about female sexuality. There are women out there in the world who, after having children and being in a long-term relationship, still pursue lots of sex.

However, in my clinic, it has been a rare woman who comes in and talks about this being a problem. Of those women who have distress around the idea of over sexuality, a fair proportion of them have been suffering different levels of mental illness. Often there are specific symptoms, such as increased sexual activity and frequent desperate masturbation with alarming daily frequency. Mental illness of course is really another subject, not in line with this book topic. There is, however, a rising trend among women to being avid solo pornography watchers and this can turn into a huge problem with guilt, shame and remorse.

It's usually the men of oversexed partners who come in with grave concerns regarding their manhood and fear they cannot keep their partner satisfied. They often feel quite bullied and coerced. It's not unlike the same reaction that women, who do not want sex have, when fervently pursued or "guilted" into having sex, which really leads us into the concept of gender role swapping. It stands to reason that for women who are lucky enough to have a high sex drive throughout their life, they might not seek the help or assistance with a counselor for that matter. I have heard of many popular blogs on the Internet about women who speak up about their high interest in sex and they want a balanced story to be made available. I commend them because the more information and personal stories we have available, the better equipped we will all be as men and women to navigate our way through life and lessen one of the biggest major lifetime stressors.

Psychological Gender or Role Swapping

This book has been mostly focused on men wanting sex constantly and women wanting emotional whole-body sex. Often in a counseling role through client dialogue, I can detect that the female actually associates much more with the emotional attributes of a man. For example, she wants uncomplicated sex, lots of it, and solves problems and doesn't listen to the man. These women are usually attracted to men who associate with more feminine attributes, such as caring for the children and wanting to discuss and share everything.

So in counseling I have to reverse my basic gender role models therapy to assist the couple work out who is whom and what they want out of the relationship. This is also true for homosexual couples. The physical gender might be the same for the partners, but their emotional gender is usually male or female predominant and relates strongly to the side of their brain they access the most in daily activities. The majority of the population is usually functioning as either right-brain thinkers exhibiting female emotions or left-brain male rationale and less emotions.

It is interesting to observe gay couples doing a dance between these two identities when they first get together. In time, they often settle on one or the other to make the balance in the coupling. Heterosexual couples also have to find a way to function in balance.

Increases Noted in Emotional Role Swapping

It would seem that in recent years an increase in changes to gender behavior have become evident. As my teenage boys grow to men, my life has been immersed in their conversations with their friends, both girls and boys. I've been fascinated watching the gender changes. I've witnessed the extreme emotional swap in girls as they pursue the young men for sex only. They phone or text, cajole and state in precise terms what they want a boy to do to them and when they want it. They have become quite demanding, seemingly with less emotion attached. In past generations, this was not so common. Girls driving on the roads are now aggressive, risk-taking and impatient. Statistics are showing more female drivers in fatalities. Even the truck-driving clients are all noticing this change in driver behavior swapping from young men to young women.

The young men are feeling awkward, pursued and definitely intimidated. Many of them are seeking emotional connections in relationships and do not behave as though they are driven and controlled by their genitalia. They are becoming badly affected when the girls ruthlessly take what they want from them and then swiftly move on to their next voyeuristic opportunity.

Perhaps this extreme swap over effect of genders is the beginning of all society coming into a balance where each person knows what it is like to be both male and female—the ultimate human—something to ponder on while you travel your life and bring up your own children.

Orgasms

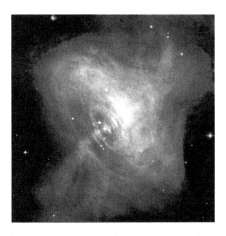

Not all women have experienced orgasm in their sexual lives or know exactly how to identify it. Perhaps this is due to the fact that there seems to be three types of orgasm most commonly felt by women and to a lesser degree by men. There is the genital orgasm, whereby the male has his orgasm through the penis and completes the process through ejaculation. The sensation of build-up forms deep in his groin region around the prostate and intensifies with a squeezing sensation until it pushes its way forward with internal spasms and release. Men naturally orgasm through ejaculation, with what could appear to be, relative ease, to a woman's mind. For a woman to reach the same relaxed mental state for orgasm to occur, many elements have to come into play when coming together as a couple.

Women who experience genital orgasms will feel these similar sensations, as they also have a small prostate, and the build-up of energy will complete its cycle through a clitoris release usually when the top aspect of the clitoris has enjoyed more stimulation. Some women can even experience ejaculation. Next, there is the vaginal release, where the vulva and clitoris will begin to squeeze tight and release multiple times. Then there is the whole body orgasm that is not usually equated or talked about as an orgasm. This experience should not be overlooked or dismissed, for it can be an experience that far exceeds the beauty and depth of feeling connected with genital climax. It is, in fact, an intense whole-body experience of beautiful spasms that seem to touch the soul. It begins by the same sexual pressure build-up in the small prostate region of the woman, but instead of making its way through the genital region, it pushes the energy upwards through the whole body via the spine. Waves of intense sheer delight reach every portion of the body, bathing the mind with a pure sense of love and connectedness. It becomes a spiritual experience. The unusual fact and gift of a whole-body orgasm is the female's ability to climax multiple times, because the energy has not dispersed out of the body via the vulva and clitoris. The sexual energy is circling through the body ready to go again and again at any time, if the right opportunity presents itself.

Sadly, for men this is not a common experience for their anatomy, but it can be practiced. Men do not have to miss out on this powerful exotic experience that touches the soul. For thousands of years the Eastern countries have had philosophies surrounding this exact experience. In India it is known as Tantric sex, coming from the study of Tantric yoga. In China, found within the ancient texts of the Taoists, there are studies and descriptions about the link between sex and longevity. The system is called Sexual Kung Fu (Kung Fu means practice) and has been mostly kept secret until a group of Taoist health practitioners came together and gifted the knowledge to the Western world.

Paramount to their philosophy is the ability for a man to enjoy complete orgasm without ejaculation. In the book, *The Multi-Orgasmic Man* by Mantak Chia and Douglas Abrams, there are step-by-step procedures to show how a man can practice this. Fortunately, the woman is not left out of the book and there is also a great section to help her. There is a special focus on how the sexual orgasmic energy can be transformed into life-giving energy that will travel to your organs providing great nourishment and strength.

This practice will increase the capacity for a couple or singles to repeatedly enjoy orgasms. These days there are many practitioners only too happy to share their knowledge, but beware, there are also some dubious ones. Many books are available that provide great information for you to explore in the privacy of your own home.

So ladies, if you have experienced anything remotely like what I have explained, then you might have had more orgasms than you realize. You do not have to accept the pressure to have a genital one. Most women I know definitely prefer the whole body scenario any day (or night) of the week, once they experience the difference between the two.

Improve Your Pleasure

Pelvic floor muscle exercises can ***improve pleasure*** and ***increase orgasm.*** When a woman has children or begins to age, usually after she reaches 30, the pelvic floor muscles begin to lose their tone. These muscles have the capacity to contract with similar strength directly related to the sensation of orgasm build-up and the actual orgasm itself. These muscles will also tighten the vaginal passage making a tighter fit for penetration, resulting in more internal friction and pleasure for the woman and external friction on the penis shaft for male stimulation. Many women are advised to do daily pelvic floor muscle or Kegel exercises (named for gynecologist Arnold H. Kegel who suggested them), especially after childbirth but also for incontinence. It is however extremely difficult to remember to fit this into an already busy schedule.

From my own experience, if you are diligent with these exercises, you will improve your sexual sensitivity. I would even say that with stronger muscles, the G-spot (named for gynecologist Ernst Gräfenberg who first described it) seems to become more accessible and easily activated. This is, of course, dependent on the exact anatomical location of that sensitive erogenous zone and will be different for everyone and might not be so simple for all women to access, but it's certainly worth a try. Even without G-spot activation, the tighter the fit, the better the friction.

For those who forget their exercises I have another solution. With research, I found a fantastic, well-reviewed product eliminating all those hours of trying to remember to attend to your daily pelvic floor health.

Lelo Luna Beads

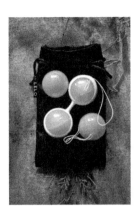

Lelo Luna Beads are the answer to help you with your pelvic floor exercises. These are a series of weighted beads that are placed in the vagina, and the woman walks around with them inside her. To prevent the balls from falling out, the woman learns to clench and tighten those important muscles of the pelvic floor. Within the small beads is another bead that moves around as you move. This slight stimulus is noted by the vagina and causes the internal muscles to react from the movement with instant contraction. So as you move, your internal muscles are working hard without your mind having to be as engaged. As your muscles become stronger, you will need to progressively step up your exercise program. With your Luna Bead purchase, there are heavier beads to do exactly that, to step up your intensity and strength. The heavier the beads are, the harder you will work to make sure they do not fall out! This is a clever system indeed!

There are many reports of increased sexual pleasure, orgasm intensity and ease of reaching these states after using the beads. Some reviewers said they used them before sex to increase sensitivity within the vagina and to create lubrication. The actual small weighted moving bead within the outside bead can at times create its own small vibration. This is why the pleasure sensations increase. They are, however, not sexual vibrators and for this reason, they not mentioned under the sex-toy section of this book.

These are available online and often found in adult shops. Some gyms and physiotherapists might also stock them.

Intensity vibrator is another product that does all the usual vibrator things, but it has two standout features that might be helpful. There is a pump section to enable the vibrator shaft to expand so that it fits tightly within. On each side of the vibrator, there are two stainless steel plates. When activated by a button, it sets off a mini electrical stimulus to make the internal muscles contract. This in effect works like a physiotherapy TENS machine but it is safe for internal use. It is the selling point of, for all intents and purposes, just another model of a vibrator. I have not been convinced with the reviews that its effect for improved pelvic floor muscles is as effective as the LELO LUNA Balls are, but it's worth a mention, especially if you think you want to explore with a vibrator. At least you will have internal muscle strengthening going on and that is a win/win situation.

Sex Toys

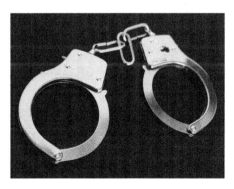

For couples these days, there is a huge onus to have an orgasm. There is so much pressure that the sex toy industry has taken off. Couples and singles everywhere are utilizing external toys to pleasure themselves or each other. For some, the use of toys feel distasteful and far removed from a sense of whole-body loving and spiritual intimate connection. Others find through the use of toys they get to know their bodies better. The reactions and sensations that can arise from different angles and the discovery of different pleasure locations within the body can be most useful to know. Later each discovery can be explored together without the use of appliances with perhaps better outcomes than before. **CAUTION:** This is however an area that can get out of control a little, if abused. Men and women might rely solely on toy use and never speak to their partner about the feeling of being let down because of the missing ingredient of whole-body intimacy. The reliance on external toys outside the natural physical connections can create even more emotional separation and distress often causing less communication.

These days there is more research about the overuse of toys and prolific masturbation with some disturbing outcomes. It has been shown that overuse of these techniques has resulted in less genital arousal over time. The body becomes desensitized by the activity and requires increased levels of stimuli and more extreme attempts to get the sexual energy arising enough for successful orgasm.

Pornography and Teens

Pornography has become quite a mainstay of sexual education among the younger generation. Explicit pictures and videos are available at the touch of a button and youngsters encounter this material more than protective parents think. When the developing minds see the images that appear, their bodies still have an uncensored reaction. The pleasure senses and chemical reactions all converge in the brain, downloading signals of desire and lustful feelings. Many youngsters, both boys and girls, report an interest in pornography and often watch it online while having sex together.

Pornography has become an early sex education for kids. They hear about sex at school and are told what physical actions take place and how pregnancy occurs, but they never cover the intimate gentle side to sex and loving that should accompany it. As the older generation, we just assume that when the younger ones experiment with sex they will naturally be showing loving kind thoughts and emotions to one another and their bodies will slowly educate them on the subtle side of loving. Not anymore!

Pornography has replaced the teacher and parent. Hardcore, same sex, dildos, three on one, anal and threesomes all become a part of the mind map created for both boys and girls around sexuality and prowess. Boys think the way you treat a porn star is how you treat your girlfriend or wife, and the girls think they have to act like a porn star to feel grunting, moaning pleasure in themselves and give great pleasure and satisfaction to their partner. This view and approach leads to disappointment, hurt, confusion and depression.

Children and young adults also think that if pornography is so easy to access, then this must be what all their parents are doing behind closed doors. Imagine those images in a child's head. They have enough problems processing normal sexual relations that parents might be having, let alone porn thoughts. Their innocent minds then sometimes ponder . . . *Is my mother being choked and taking it up the butt right now? Is my dad choking Mom and urinating on her? Is that what I am expected to accept as a woman when I am married?* The boy might be thinking, *How can I fit my fist up there? Is my dad doing that to my mom? Girls like it like that and it's normal.*

These are never good images for a developing mind to have to process. This arena of pornography I am finding in the clinic has become the new sexual abuse of our generations. Girls are scared of and loathing sex. Boys are also scared because they have to speak dirty horrible words toward the girl they feel love for. If he doesn't, she might think he is useless as a male by not providing porn-style loving. Our education has to go further.

I have had to listen to stories of widowed or divorced women who tell of their regretful sexual encounters with younger men. At first, they think it's exciting to go to check out the nightclubs and have some muscled young man make sexual approaches to them. They take the risk and go home with the young lad. Before she knows it, they are one moment kissing, and the next minute she is bent over and has a penis violently stuck up her anus. Suddenly feeling violated, mortified and scared she goes off her head and berates the boy. He is confused, apologetic and doesn't know what he did wrong. He did not know that intimacy and trust are usually established first before adventures in the back playground might ever even be considered.

This newer generation of porn viewers is also creating a lot of video footage of themselves that often ends up being shared in inappropriate ways. Revenge tactics of a jilted partner can really turn ugly and are a great cause behind severe depression and suicide.

It is more important than ever that parents take it on themselves to be more open and explain the difference between pornographic sex and loving sex. The young adults need more guidance in these matters than has been done in the past. So I beseech parents to take a big step and start talking openly about pornography.

Pornography and Couples

Many couples, as they struggle to come to terms with their lagging sexual relationship, might decide to try using pornography to stimulate the situation. Men who are stimulated visually will quickly embrace this idea often encouraging their partner toward this solution. It suits their needs. Women who are desperate to please their partner, who are guilt-ridden or secretly bored sexually by their partner, might also be keen to try this and explore sexual toys together.

From conversations, it seems that women can become quite excited visually also for a time and the pornography pathway works. Then the female mind that craves love and connectedness takes over and all the visual stimulation systematically switches off the body senses and the woman is relegated back to square one. She returns to her inner paranoia and guilt. A new cycle begins, potentially into new levels of experimentation.

Often, in the back of the female mind, is the idea that the man is getting off more on the images on the screen than the togetherness she is so desperately trying to recreate by participating in these adventures. This troubles her deeply, yet she keeps trying to please him, often at the detriment of her own inner self worth, many times triggering depression. When the man shows such obvious joy and intensity in the pornographic material, doubt about the long-term intimacy of the relationship inevitably follows.

When women pursue sexual release through sex toys, great experiences can be had, but they are all surrounding an isolated physical orgasm that is vastly separated from the whole-body infused loving when two people merge together in mutual love/lust- making. The pursuit of sheer physical release can get rid of pent-up forces until even that becomes boring and disconnected. Humans crave connectedness with one another. Even men crave being intimately close to a living, breathing partner rather than just a life of masturbation and sex toys. If a man can be satisfied only with the physical release, then he would just use his hand and never need to pursue and engage with another person. Each gender has the DNA to procreate, which requires the human physical connection to one another.

On a positive note, some couples engaging sexually while watching pornography confirm that it has helped and repaired their sex life. This is due to their communication improving and the woman finding the courage to talk more openly and demonstrate what feels nice for her. Some of her initial shyness has been replaced with a deeper confidence in her own body and she feels better understood by her partner.

Neural Networking of the Brain

Current research in neuroscience is discovering some alarming statistics about brain function and the capacity for the brain to become conditioned. When the brain receives stimuli, over and over again of the same material, it eventually normalizes and no longer responds in an excited state. The release of happy chemicals does not occur as the brain is now trained and bored. It needs a new higher stimulus of pornography to get the same reactions. This is the story of pornography addiction. The images have to become more hard-core and violent to get the responsive sexual high. Porn addicts, both men and women, have to deal with this problem. If a man cannot become stimulated by his normal partner because she is not behaving and accepting sexual behavior like a porn star, then it becomes boring and causes impotence. Women often experience less lubrication effects or any heightened sexual interest in their relationship. Shame, guilt, distress and broken marriages result.

When these ill effects are noted after the adventures have

soured, then new layers of emotional distress often creep into the relationship, not to mention the individual mind. This damage will need professional counseling to unravel.

Warning on Threesomes, Wife Swapping and Sex

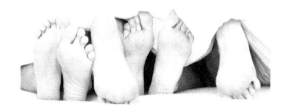

It has often amused me when some heterosexual females, married with kids, suddenly announce they are gay. Not because of their life-altering announcement, but how they suddenly know this about themselves. Some of them when I ask them how they discovered this, they mentioned they finally, after much pressure from their partner and living with guilt and shame about a low sex drive, ended up in a threesome—two females with one male.

The result of this adventure was the woman loved the emotional connection she made with the other woman and dumped her husband, much to his shock and horror. He thought all his birthdays had come at once to have this opportunity to be with two women at the same time. So beware, men—do not underestimate the desperate need for a woman to feel loved completely. The introduction of another woman might provide the necessary ingredients that you are lacking and before you know it, you find yourself in the divorce courts.

This same issue can also happen with the two-male/one-female partnering. Your male partner might have a strong emotional connection enough to not leave you for the other man, but he might discover he's turned on by the adventure and wants to pursue it again. Sometimes the threesome includes you, but many times he might take it on himself to pursue the bisexual adventures on his own.

If it's not sexual orientation that challenges the relationship, it might be that the partner falls in love/ lust with the third person and a separate relationship is pursued outside of the open arrangements. This is a common occurrence with couples I have counseled under these situations. What started out as fun, exciting and voyeuristic quickly falters and transforms into distrust, jealousy and separation.

Think about what doors you want opened and explored in your life before you take action.

The swingers clubs involving couples going to dinner and throwing the keys in the middle and swapping sex with one another is another pastime for some. This makes fertile ground for secret affairs developing outside of the club activities. Once both of you agree to let others participate in your joint intimacy and commitment, you are potentially calling in complex webs of danger. Think before you act or accept new relationship parameters. Decide what you want out of life and who you want to be. What are your personal value systems? Do you have the courage to find emotional support if it all goes terribly wrong?

With all these scenarios, there are potentially more alarming outcomes that might have not initially been understood or expected. It has mostly concerned me when women have come to my clinic or phoned me and they are absolutely devastated by the choices of partner swapping. They are revolted and ashamed at themselves for being so easily coerced into this as a pathway to resolve the inner conflict with sex and intimacy. They have only agreed because of the fear of losing their partner to others. They grasp and hold on to the hope that these new decisions will fix the problem and they will gain acceptance and non-judgment from the partner. Sadly, most of their minds and hearts turn in on themselves and they find themselves in a hole they cannot dig out of.

Essentially, through their decision, they become a sexual victim and perpetrator to themselves. They also view their partner in the same light—respect vanishes, love is eaten up. They are left with feelings of shame, guilt, feeling dirty, lonely and powerless. Serious therapy is required, and most often these people leave the current relationship, moving on to a whole new level of personal emotional baggage and wariness.

Sex and Drugs

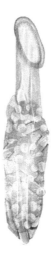

Many clients are slow to admit they use drugs. When they have felt comfortable enough with me, they open up to their exploration of substance abuse. This might be in the form of alcohol, marijuana, ecstasy tablets or even harder drugs. Stories are related of the substances helping them to loosen up to the idea of sex with their partner when they otherwise might not be inclined or the body just does not get turned on anymore.

In these instances substances become the new relationship rescue. A person often feels like it's the only way they can keep the interest of their partner. This thought process is evident with women. They will risk their own health and well-being just to keep the intimate connection with a partner for fear they will be abandoned and another partner will take their place. Sadly, serious addiction creeps in without knowing how to get off the moving train.

From consistent comments I receive, marijuana seems to increase the body sensations and sensitivity, and the genital regions experience more blood flow and therefore heightened sexual enjoyment. I've known people who have sensibly used "weed" for this purpose without addiction, but there are others who have not fared so well. I believe the added effects of drugs on the body in relation to sexual activity is worthy of far more research and exploration about a connection to the increased explosion of drug use in this world.

Alcohol is commonly used to help people face their relationship problems. I don't even like using the word, "help," as I really think it ultimately hinders the process of life and reality. My concern for people going on this path of exploration is the temptation to cover up underlying issues, just for the sake of some emotional reprieve from anxiety about sexuality and their relationships. It is my experience with people in therapy that you can only cover up deep underlying issues for so long before the issue arises from the subconscious, presenting all the same issues as before. So it's far better to face the problem head on and delve into why you feel the way you do. I'm hoping this book might shed light and hope on those women and men who think they have to take such extreme measures in order to continue to live life joyfully with a partner.

Why Do Men Choose Prostitutes?

Now this is not a subject that most women would like to think about, as there is a lot of fear around the idea of prostitution and paying for sex. There are quite a few reasons why men or women might choose to hire the services of someone in this profession. Predominantly men might be the usual clientele but with the increased rate of pornography viewing, couples might be choosing higher levels of experimentation in the safety of anonymity.

When speaking to women of the prostitution profession, I actually find that a large proportion of men who attempt to use the service, end up sitting on the bed, uncomfortable to disrobe and just want to talk. Their issues might well be ones of loneliness; starved for affection or human touch; a partner who ignores, refuses to listen or is consumed by demands of children, family and friends; any issues of the above leave them feeling no longer a viable part of the relationship equation. They exist in the home, not as an alpha male, but as a working servant with little appreciation thrown their way. It might have taken them 20 years to cross the threshold of a sex worker's parlor door, but eventually the loss of self-identity drives them.

Many sex workers fulfill a vital role in the community that regular wives might not. Fantasies can be acted out, the ease of speaking up for needs and specific touch is much easier if you're paying for a service. The capacity to fill a role of counseling where services might be lacking should not be underestimated. A man going to counseling appears weak. Going to a prostitute is cool and acceptable. Their friends will never know if they acted on the service or not.

In Asia, the sex trade is huge and obviously fills a need in society. When you walk the night streets in Thailand, you'll always see the male tourists loving the generous attention lavished on them.

The Asian women fill a really special niche. Men and women get to chat, laugh and play board games for many hours as the bar girls giggle, pat and stroke and compliment their potential clientele.

Not all men who frequent these places are lonely. Many have wives and families to go home to. They could be consistent philanderers and adulterers, sex addicts, closet bisexuals or homosexuals and just need to find an outlet. Some will be hesitant husbands, but the doting, open, honest invitation from Asian women becomes too hard for a rational mind to assess the potential damage. Feeling a desperate need to feel loved and cared for and treated like a king can really push a man over the edge toward these promising Asian smiles.

The love affair men have with Asian women is their absolute femininity and delicate bodies. It makes the men feel strong, virile, powerful and protective—all qualities that men love within themselves. They love to feel those emotions being accepted and played out. In the Western world, women often take over the role of being male and female—a virtual Amazon woman. Through their desperate need for equality and acknowledgment, this might have gone too far for a good relationship. It would be remiss of me to not factor the issue of over burdened financial commitments forcing women to join the ranks of male workers often leaving the alpha male stranded and alone trying to find his own position of importance. If it's not through work then he looks for his sense of value and appeal elsewhere.

Sometimes when men partner with a delicate, feminine woman who refuses to do any male-type activities, he quickly tires. He becomes bored with changing light bulbs, climbing stepladders for high objects or cutting back bushes. He sees a woman as perfectly able to do these things herself. His love affair of petite and needy withers and dies. Men might love to make love to a feminine woman but they love their long-term partner to be a companion, closely resembling male friendships.

So ladies, if you want to minimize the risk of a man straying and having his needs met elsewhere, then you need to step up the antics. Be gentle and feminine and attentive, cook the meals, wash the clothes, and treat him like a king. Start sex by being gentle, then BANG! Go hard at it! Don't nag him to do anything that he thinks you should do yourself, whatever that is, then hang out and help him with his interests like a good friend. Simple? Hmmmm . . . We can all choose which parts of that advice we can live with. I know it's never as simple as that, but still worth pondering.

Just remember—when you engage the services of another person in the intimate areas of your life, you have introduced a third party into your relationship, and complications usually follow. Think before you leap.

Celia Fuller

{ 6 }
Life Gets in the Way

Partners Working Away

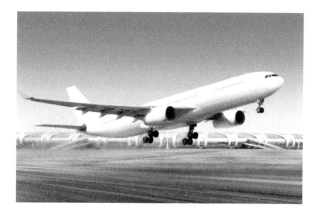

As our world becomes smaller with the advent of affordable air flight, more people are traveling and working away for long periods of time. Military personnel, miners, air attendants, building con-tractors and all their support personnel are called upon to spend larger amounts of time away from family to fulfill the constant rise in the cost of living, or position themselves in higher roles.

These huge efforts are admirable but can come at a cost to the relationship and family life that men and women are trying to sustain. It's when they come home that they realize something has changed. Their fantasies of returning to a sex-thirsty female might be drastically altered, instead finding their partner distant, disconnected and in no rush for the bedroom. If you're a female returning home, you're probably hanging out for a cup of tea and a shower, only to encounter your sex-starved man waiting in fer-vent hope for a wild lustful episode.

So what goes wrong? Here's the problem—when a man leaves the family home, the woman must shut up shop sexually. With that comes a shutting down of her intimate emotional self, placing a large wall around herself so no intruders dare come near. Knowing she'll feel pain and loss, she works furiously at a subconscious level to bury all her feelings that loving someone brings. As a month drags on, she has been forced to get on with life by not having to consider the partner's need in any way, shape or form. Slowly the memory of intimacy dims to an idea, not so much fact. Women don't usually have the same daily supercharged sexual energy that keeps reminding them, so she buries those feelings.

If she's the mother of children, she's had to take on two roles: one of nurturing mother and the other as disciplinarian father. New family rules and regulations are implemented that help the mother keep the home front in order, as now she has no backup. She must cope, as she has no other choice. The kids have to adapt. Some of her rules might not make sense to the missing man, but they work for her just so she can get by and manage.

So when the man comes home, two issues arise. First, the woman is cold and emotionally distant, programmed to keep all the men away. She might feel lusting situations within her body, but to race into intimacy is incredibly difficult. For women to open themselves to sexual loving, one must first remove the barrier. This takes time and requires women to feel and be in the presence and personality of her partner for a while before her defenses come down.

If a man pushes past that defense too fast, without respecting the woman's needs and feelings, then the woman might feel abused, even if she sometimes accept the advances. Mostly women are dutiful and know what is expected, but it's one thing to act on the expectation and another to think and feel quite differently. If there are negative feelings or emotions associated with the sexual encounter, then those feelings become buried and fester without ever verbalizing them, often not even recognizing the problem. This is due to it being a duel experience that involves, excitement, knowing we will see our loved one but dread at what is to unfold and especially how soon intimacy will be expected. Single women have the same issues, except their sexuality is often much harder to put on hold and wait. Their sexual energy issues have not usually decreased at this stage unless they are in a long-term relationship.

Imagine the poor man's devastation to not find a sex-starved partner waiting for him. He is surely sex-starved and possibly in pain with "blue-ball syndrome." He can't wait to have a release that is not given by his own hand. He wants to be loved and feel loved and gift his loving partner immediately with no delay. That is his welcome back home, making working away so much more worthwhile.

Male Hints to Ease Transition When Coming Home

Number One. Don't criticize changes in furniture, decor or family rules. There is plenty of time to tackle those items and being negative serves no one, since you'll be away from home soon enough and it won't affect you unless your wage is being sucked dry. Now that will be an issue. Criticism puts another defensive layer on a woman's wall of emotional disconnect. Words of disapproval only activate negative feelings and are not considered foreplay. You should be open, receptive and observant. Take some time to settle in. Hug, hold and gently kiss—no leaping tongues gouging the tonsils out, just genuine pleasure to be home and let your partner know you missed her. Remember, they need to feel like a person, not a sexual object.

If you play a little hard-to-get, you might even raise some curiosity. There is a possibility that you might be accused of playing up if you hold back, but if you allow just enough proof that you love them then those anxieties will settle. Rest assured that in most cases women will be hanging out for their bodies and minds to get with the program and enjoy you fully. It just takes more time, potentially more time than a shower and a Full Monty parading the house showing your need. The truth is, women all report that this process can take a couple of days. They experience your return home as though you were almost a stranger, and they are not ready to be handled, tongue-groped or your seed implanted on day one. There is a customization period.

When I talk to women, most of them cannot even put these conflicting feelings into words. They live with anxiety undressed and a nagging, doubting dread stirs within, feeding their brain with fearful thoughts of not loving their partner any more. By day three they suddenly realize they do, but another layer of resentment might have been added if the man pushed his affections too soon and made her feel forced and coerced into activities not of her own mind.

These psychological shifts and changes can really hold a relationship in a precarious sense of balance. If a woman can understand this about herself then she can also help the man accept and feel welcomed home.

What Can a Woman Do for a Man In This Situation?

Remember, he's had to leave you with visions of making your joint life better. He doesn't know that his decision might result in such confusing messages when he comes home. Knowing he's returning home to love, he'll work his heart out using work to suppress his sexual urges. While he's away on any time off, his mind will be plagued by beautiful memories that always end up with him feeling horny. He might take his needs into his own hands, so to speak, just for initial peace, but it never replaces the whole-body loving and emotional connection to a partner.

When he leaves, he can often feel great guilt and worry for your safety. He hangs out daily to come home to you and the home you've created together. This is the place he does not have to prove himself, because you accept him as he is. Loving kindness is what they ask for and consideration for all their efforts, so what can you do when he comes home?

Kiss quickly, hug, hold and don't give him a cup of tea or a beer, otherwise you'll immediately go into nervous chatty mode like a girlfriend has arrived and spend hours catching up on all that has gone on since he was away. I know it's tempting. He can't listen properly anyway, as his mind is dealing with much more urgent matters. He'll get restless and short with you. Instead, send him in to have a shower and surprise him with a frothy hand job! Tend his needs, give him a release and then he'll wait less grumpily for you to have time to let your intimate walls down.

Now the man might feel confused and a little put off by the instant offer of a hand job, considering he has been away for a long time, while in his imagination he has been thinking about making love to you completely. So it is important that you explain how much you love him, buts it's difficult to open up so quickly to make love and you are offering this as a simple way to begin reconnecting.

As I've said before, you'll be amazed at the transformation. It's all about understanding each other and listening to each other's needs. Communicate, explore, play and take action to see what works for you.

Changing Authority Figures

Number Two. The second issue is when a man comes home to a family of children. He left home entrusting his partner with nurturing, maintaining rules, and managing the home in the way they jointly negotiated or how one might have dictated. With the choice to work away, often you have released the right to a fair degree of your parenting authority. You handed the baton to your partner with unsaid words of trust. You stepped out and away, allowing them to use their full discretion in family life, perhaps not realizing how much harder life would be as a single parent, juggling all the complexities of home life, children's education and sporting activities without emotional backup. There is no hugging or holding to say they're doing a great job, instead they might be experiencing sneaking resentment for the free life you are supposedly enjoying.

So when you come home, don't jump on the kids, roaring and reprimanding them about broken rules. This will only cause your partner to feel unappreciated, bossed, rejected and protective of her environment she had to create while you were away. She has been mostly doing the best she can under the circumstances. Don't make her feel as if life is easier without you in it, by your need to exert your alpha male placement in the home. Your children will also feel traumatized and shocked by you bursting their bubble of routine. They also have had to go through grief and loss and constant adapting to you coming and going in their lives. Be gentle; take time to know everyone again.

If you've been away a month, then everyone in your life has changed just as you have changed. Your partner might have been forced to develop resilience and a sense of accomplishment—something not felt before. So with you away, you've gifted her an opportunity to grow in confidence. She just might have taken a liking to being the solo boss with the family settling to a different rhythm.

The children too have finally settled, getting used to you not coming in the door every day. They have learned to defer to your partner as the overruling parent. Your role has been usurped, your castle taken over. Taking over does not bode well if done by force.

WARNING: If you jump on the kids and unsettle them, the mother hen will peck your eyes out and there will be no sex on the menu. You serve no one with this approach. Return home with gentleness of spirit, quietly sit among the family, play with the children and read them books. This is what helps you get laid. Get to the woman through loving her children. Yes, they are your children too, but while you've been away, they've been HER children.

When you talk, play and listen, she'll want to join in and sit near you. As the gentleness and your open awareness of your changing family needs unravel, she will feel a change come over her. Easier affection will reveal her walls gently falling down, allowing you to be in her most sacred intimate space again. If she does not join you because she's busy, encourage her to leave the work for a few moments. These are the insights that can change the whole family dynamic. No one wants World War III in his or her living room. Let the dust settle on your arrival first. Allow the delights to follow.

In the last section, I focused on the man being the only one away from home and then returning. If you are the woman returning, the picture is not so different. You will have your walls up, and he will be waiting at home with an eager erection. If you can get that sorted after a hug, kiss and all-important cup of tea, shower and talk to the kids, then you will give yourself the essential time you need to adapt being back on the home front.

Having kids and finding time for your partner is really difficult but, ladies, you can make your life easier by this approach. Just don't spoil them too much. They still have to also jump to some of your tunes.

A mother can also feel like the boss of the home because, even though she's been away, her psycho-observation skills will pick up so many things a man might have overlooked. She will jump on them with precision and leap into the role of taking over all the activities at the home front, also unsettling the dynamics. A man might easily step aside and say, "Here, have it, go your hardest," but there will still be a little resentment and criticism. So you too must move back into the space with gentleness.

Why Can Women Scream at the Kids, but Men Can't?

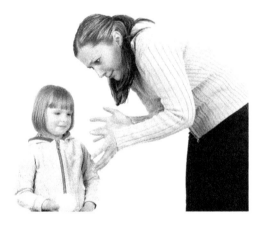

Criticizing the children is like criticizing the marriage. At a deep level within a woman's heart, children are a representation of the marriage. Unknown to them, they gauge the health of the marriage by how well the children are treated by the male. If she notes aggression and criticism, she will immediately feel the rise of temper, offense and even personal wounding. The male will become Enemy No. 1 and all forces of the female's arsenal will be directed at him to make him stop.

It's a strange phenomenon, but when I bring this up with women in counseling conversations, it's as if a light flicks on. When I ask a woman, "Why is it ok for you to yell and scream irrationally at the kids with a barrage of distressing comments, but when the man does it, you jump down his throat?" You don't tolerate their actions and you accuse him of not loving the kids, hurting and damaging their feelings. He's completely confused by the turn of events, has no idea why he gets the silent treatment, especially when he was backing up your irrational rant of only moments before, yet you act as though your behavior is ok but his is not.

For the logical male mind, this is insanity. This behavior is completely irrational until you understand that, to a woman, she reacts to a man as though he is yelling at her, not the kids, and verbalizing his dissatisfaction with her. She decides to take on those feelings of wounding because she is still trying to work through some of her own emotional feelings that are not sitting well with her.

If you listen to the words she uses, there will be hidden keys to what is going on in her innermost subconscious world about the relationship. This is a chance for men to step up, listen and support. When you are loving the children, you are loving the marriage. How you react to the children is also a reflection of the marriage from the females subconscious perspective. Women, give the men a break. They don't know this about your reactions either. All of this information is new to them, as much as it is to you. With knowledge comes awareness; with awareness comes communication and acceptance. We are all growing in this whirlpool of life.

Grief—Abortions, Adoptions and Child Death

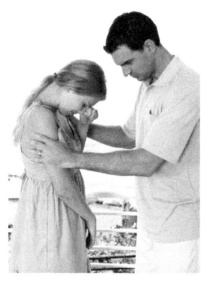

The grief cycle a woman goes through with any event involving the loss of a child occurs in an intense way. It's not just for a couple of days or a month, it sits with her Being, cradled forever, and remembered like a burning cauldron. She might have learned to keep on living, but the anguish rises to the surface in a perpetual cycle. She values the memory of a child's life, no matter how small a time she had with him or her. She values and listens to the way her child changed her. The child is part of her journey that cannot be buried and pushed aside.

In my experience in a clinical setting, men most often also feel a dramatic sense of loss, but their rational, logical minds see no reason to talk about it. They know they are powerless to change the loss and they know they must just keep living through the pain. The only way they know how to survive the emotions is to push them as far away from the mind as they possibly can. Emotions make them feel out of control. They fear them and they run from them. That is how they survive. They do not know how to support a woman who must continually anguish about it.

Sometimes a man's suppressed pain makes them sick, as they've had to harden their hearts just to keep going. The pain sits underneath the surface, like a brewing volcano. Women want to feel pain in every memory cell of the body as though she is a living memorial because from within her body, the spark of a new creation began life. She has cherished and nurtured every second, every day since conception. Her body has ensured survival until it could no longer. Guilt and failure often invade her mind. She tries to overcome this, but she always honors the memory. She comes to understand herself, her environment and the future by the way she conducts herself through loss. She cannot grasp that a man does not carry his heart on his sleeve as she does. Resentment and hurt follow.

Warning Bells in a Relationship, Dealing With Loss

Women lose respect for a man in a huge way when they don't grieve in the same fashion as they do. They accuse the man of being callous, hard, uncaring and even a sense of being betrayed by them can arise. Betrayed because they believe something about the man that ended up not being true. She thinks that he did not feel the same level of care and love and loss as she did because he is grieving differently. Rest assured, ladies, they grieve as much as you do.

I have seen so many relationships fall apart due to the grieving loss of a child, no matter how it happened or what stage of development the child was at—in vitro or walking and talking. When a man cannot find the words to explain how he feels because pain is too much to bear, he risks alienating the love of his life, his partner. She does not cope with the silence and takes to heart that he must not care. It is really difficult for her to find peace around the man's opposite reactions and focus and his ability to move on. When she feels such opposition to this, she'll close all her communication channels, sex being the first to go. There is no energy left to nourish the person who she believes is callous and heartless.

Men, you need to find a new way of listening and allowing your grieving partner to talk. Her grief will rise and fall, mostly she'll seek her own counsel to process but she will need to know that you still remember the child—that you also, in your most private hours, think about all that happened. You have to let her know, because if she believes she's living a lie with you and feels betrayed, it will eat up all the goodness from the relationship. She might take her body and her living memories away from you and you'll no longer have access to her feelings that secretly help you through yours. Lead her into your heart, allow her to feel and share your pain. She will then know she is not struggling alone. The fears of being misunderstood and alone are the ingredients of relationship breakdown, depression and health complaints.

Sexual Affairs /Emotional Affairs

There are two types of affairs—the sexual affair and the emotional affair. Now we all know that for a partner to make a choice to have sexual affair with another person can be extremely hurtful and usually ends the relationship. Or so one would think from the media. This happens in many cases, but there are equally as many people who try really hard to push through those acts of betrayal and create a new version of their life together.

SEXUAL AFFAIRS: Men, no matter how hard they try, often cannot get past the fact that another male has parked his penis within a woman who he thinks of as his. Because they think in pictures, this image usually invades their mind quite often. Anger also becomes a number one emotion because the woman has probably rejected his advances on many, many occasions, and he was led to believe she did not want sex. He has suffered emotional failure and passed up numerous offers from other girls to only have this outcome as his reward. Often that is where a betrayal takes up home and becomes the destructive power for the relationship. Not often does a man think about the emotional connection that a woman might have felt for the man.

Women, on the other hand, really don't like the thought of their partner with another woman, but it's how the man has reacted within the affair that grieves the woman the most. *What sweet words did he tell her? What has he promised to her that keeps her waiting for him? What has he said about me? Has he done all the things with her that he never would with me? Did he secretly take her dancing or wining and dining while at home he chooses to fester on the couch? Did other people see him loving it up as he brazenly showed the world his loving connection? Did they walk arm in arm or hand in hand, as he displayed his sense of pride to walk by her side?* Thoughts and imaginings, such as these eat away at her core, and even though she might try to get over those deep thoughts of doubt, they arise time and time again.

The sexual act of her spouse with another woman is secondary where the woman is concerned. Her thoughts then become extended to the bedroom. *Did he roll over and go to sleep after sex with her? Or did he stroke, cuddle and hold her, murmuring sweet talk in her ears? Did they laugh and frolic as lustful teens behind closed doors, while she was at home with screaming children or sulky teens, yearning desperately for anything that looked like that kind of freedom.*

Its thoughts such as these that torture the female mind and if this has happened in your relationship, you will be sure it will have an impact on your future lovemaking, if you decide to keep your current relationship alive. A lot of patience and reassurance will need to be gently exerted while being vigilant to your own weaknesses. Those exact weaknesses are the areas that can be explored with counseling support and should be, if you want to have any chance at the relationship moving healthily forward.

EMOTIONAL AFFAIRS: Never underestimate the power that an emotional affair can have on a woman. As a man, you might claim that you never had sex with the person but just talked and liked the other's company. So, therefore, you are innocent of any wrongdoing and cannot understand why you are experiencing the wrath of your partner. Women can cope with their spouse having a general chat with other women, as that is normal among friend's wives and their friends. It's when the personal, emotional sharing starts to become intensive that the wife or partner will start having some kind of insecure reaction.

This feeling of insecurity and resentment comes from the man not usually opening up and freely chatting at home to their partner. For most women to get any open communication at home, it's like pulling teeth. So when they know the man is at the office and lunching with the same female or multiple females or connecting to a woman in a greater way, they begin to feel angry. Women will give anything to have the communication and laughter in their relationship return, but they don't know what to do or how to help get it back. So when a man seems to respond by sharing his deepest thoughts, wishes and dreams with someone else, often with a dose of manly flirting and complimenting, it can be experienced as a major betrayal. Not everyone would see it this way, but it does come up a lot in counseling as the woman begins to imagine the worst of her partner as his behavior drives home her inadequacies, which activates her fears and phobias.

These insecurities can stop any bedroom activity overnight, because she is never sure if he has actually crossed the line with the woman. Her internal grief consumes her and the man has no idea what is going on. His behaviors might well be innocent at that stage, not even knowing the dangerous game he is playing. In his mind (if he has even thought it), he is getting his emotional needs met by someone who seems to value him and has not spent the last 10 years or so nagging or sexually rejecting him.

Emotional affairs can quickly turn into sexual ones for both sexes. If you are a man reading this and you are enjoying the company of other women, perhaps what you really need is to speak to a professional and get your needs met in a safe environment. Then use that to benefit the relationship, nourish the partnership, help each other grow and feel loved, valued, important and above all respected.

So far, I have just focused on the man having an emotional or sexual affair. Let's now address the woman.

Women and affairs are a complicated situation. Men can feel threatened by other men showing increased attention to their partner. They know exactly what is formulating in the male mind and it's not good. A man might not comment to the woman about these hidden fears or warn her that some of her behavior could be considered sexual encouragement from a male perspective.

Women don't usually allow affairs to happen easily and they occur usually after long thought. Spontaneous sexual decisions might be made, but usually the woman has already fantasized a lot about any man coming into her life who has all the characteristics that her partner no longer exhibits. If the right man appears, fitting her needs, then she will often just walk out of the relationship not being able to withstand her own inner sense of wrongdoing and normal integrity levels. A woman can just have sex and leave it at that, but more often than not, if they enjoy more than one encounter with the same person, emotional links begin to form. If the emotional links form, then the woman will usually leave the current relationship regardless of having someone to run to. She will just leave and start a new life. Many men, on the other hand, seem to be able to separate their external sex encounters from their committed home relationship and still function well.

Please be aware these are generalizations of the genders and I have seen many different and unusual choices with couples as they navigate their various ways to try to understand themselves. It is not easy and it is fraught with hidden barriers and potholes. Affairs can often arise from much deeper psychological wounds, trauma and conditioning that might be reinventing itself and exerting its influence on current choices. It is for this reason that support really should be sought to help you with those **impulsive feelings.**

Magnetic Attraction

Magnetic attractions are the most dangerous of all. Temptations can arise from an insane magnetism experienced by two people who may be strangers to each other. It's like sex at first sight as two minds seem to combine, skipping the physical stages. This is one situation where all logic or rational thinking can be overtaken by an impulse of attraction that has no rhyme or reason. Fantasies are born from this space as the magnitude of feelings drive those two people into each other's arms.

When ignited by this fire all other loved ones are usually pushed aside as the person attempts to process what might be happening to them. These attractions can quickly move from the emotional affair stage to sexual affair before they even have a chance to really think before acting or assessing what they are risking. Male and females can both be victims to such chance meetings and will have to be very quick in salvaging their sanity before they cross the line from promise and commitment, to intoxicating exploration. I believe every relationship will have at least one of these chance meetings during their relationship. It is the ultimate challenger and relationship changer.

The concepts of Soul Mates, or finding their other half, are often the thoughts surrounding the idea of magnetic attraction.

Celia Fuller

{ 7 }
Psychological Barriers Inhibiting Intimacy

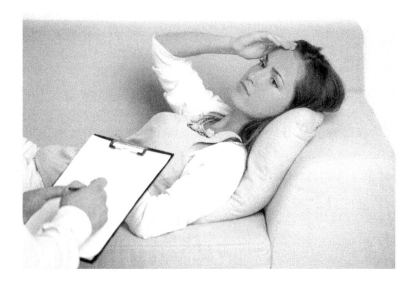

Emotional Mental Patterning and Conditioning

So far we've explored the opposite gender reactions and needs to live a life of contentment around sexuality. Often it can be a simple problem and with a few adjustments, life manages to maintain an even keel. If only it was that simple. As humans, together on this planet, we need to exercise so much more awareness around the emotional mental patterns of others and ourselves. Knowledge with gentleness will really help uncover the true cause behind some of the worst relationship issues that arise in a lifetime.

So for this next chapter, I will share with you many scenarios that might directly impact your sexual life or that of your partner. It is my hope that this will help open the dialogue for you both to explore more deeply the subconscious reason behind actions, reactions and thought processes, as events from the past are known to impact and map out your behavior in the future. Whatever you experience in early life ends up implanting within your subconscious later revealing itself in strange actions, behaviors, and mutated emotional responses, all affecting your potential to find joy and harmony in life.

When you decide to make a change in your life, you need to explore the hidden aspects and memories within the subconscious so those events that have a negative impact on you can be changed and overcome. Each person in a relationship must honor and respect the other and help facilitate this personal journey of discovery, and who knows, you might even have more sex, possibly even better earthshaking intimate sex with passion and empathy.

Effects of Sexual Abuse

One of the single most sexually debilitating experiences for people is sexual abuse at a young age. This also involves nonconsensual touching and taking advantage of a young confused mind that seems to be consensual but does not even know what they are consenting to as they are coerced into something.

If a person is violently sexually abused as a child, he or she will live life feeling horror, shame and guilt at their secret, and repulsion at physical contact with others when deep intimacy is required. This might not be evident straightaway as love-lust has a power beyond itself to keep these feelings and memories hidden. It is a soothing balm to a wounded heart. However, as a relationship continues, there are more opportunities for the deeper memories and subsequent emotional reactions to become triggered and surface, thus creating behaviors of sexual aversion, non-safety, terror and fear of punishment.

Another unusual scenario can play out as sexual addiction behavior. If a female child is sexually abused in the past by her father in a secretive coercing loving way, then she might create a belief that to recreate that feeling of intense, secretive fatherly love then she must instigate sexual activity with any man she feels a connection with. Often this overt sexual behavior occurs at an early age due to the child's desperation to feel a sense of security and connection.

On the other hand, the child might not seek it out, but could associate with feelings of fear and punishment if he or she doesn't obey. So any time the developing young boy or girl has someone older or in power demanding sex or suggesting it, then they might feel powerless to say, "no, stop." In fear of the punishment threat that has been embedded in their earlier memories, sometimes it might look to others like behaviors of sexual addiction and that they love it. In truth, the total opposite might be true.

There is also a strong link to homosexuality, especially among girls, due to the dire consequences of forced sexual abuse on the girl child and her trust issues toward men that have been shattered. The inner dialogue could sound something like this:

- Man is a beast—cruel, hurtful—I cannot trust men, they are savage with no personal emotional touching.
- The only people I feel safe with are women. They are the same as me, so I know my feelings and reactions toward sex and therefore they are female, so I am safe.

The women might be strongly attracted to men, but they cannot take sex to intimate levels. If they do, every part of their psychological Being, screams with alarm.

Sometimes these behaviors, feelings and connections are

obvious all through life, however, it is a huge confusing surprise if these feelings never arise until you've found a partner who might actually be quite similar in small ways to the perpetrator and the next thing you know memories are activated.

Men who have been abused as children, especially as youth, might have experienced genital pleasure from the abuse if it was not enacted in a severe way. If they felt pleasure, but it was mixed with shame and aversion to the same-sex event, they can have raging doubts about their sexuality. I've come across this a lot in a clinical setting. Men have been anguished all their lives with the terrible secret—the fear they might be gay. The reasoning behind this is because, as they were abused, their body parts had a reaction, even when their emotions were screaming the opposite. They fear that one day their secret will be discovered and their female partner will not understand.

In fact, on many occasions this has been a correct fear, because women do not understand the sheer sensitivity of the male appendage. Women cannot believe a man is not capable of stopping an erection, if touched a certain way, or halting his subsequent ejaculation. For the young teen, who's filled with grief and mind-dementing shame that the body betrayed his own mind, he lives with that, worries about it, and yet has no one to talk with about it. This shame can eat away at his ability to have open, loving sex with a partner, because he's holding a deep secret inside.

Unexpected Erections

So strong is the sexual impulse in men that erections often activate during fight-and-flight situations. So when violent sexual abuse is evident, so too is the fight/flight survival of the species sexual orientation activated. The fear of imminent death and harm will activate a male system to release sperm in order to procreate. This sudden onset of an erection can confuse boys and young teens who have been sexually abused. They often will feel guilt, shame and live in fear that part of their anatomy behaved in a manner that might have appeared as encouragement to the degenerate act, thus causing many psychological problems later on in their lives. Even a nervous fear response will activate these sensations and sexual drive. Hearing this from a female's perspective, it really must be a curse to be a male with this as a problem.

Other stories I've heard are of tales of musicians who before going on stage have wild erections, sometimes to the point of needing to masturbate to make their appendage behave on stage! So too have I read and heard many counts of men in military situations who have been forced to deal with raging, mind-numbing erections while trying to deal with being in combat mode. Some accounts I've read of Vietnam veterans have been the horror and shame they experienced when they became a sexual perpetrator in the time of war and they enacted behaviors they never would have done if their lives were not threatened. Many commit suicide. They cannot live with their actions. After war, their fight/flight adrenalin is often never fully turned off. Their minds and thinking drive them insane and they can never trust their own potential behaviors.

Men in war are not alone with this happening. Women in war also become highly sexed, as the animal part of their brain is driven to perpetuate the species. There is no physical rhyme or reason. I remember a story of a soldier and a nurse, unknown to each other, throwing themselves into a wild sexual act out in the open up against a building while bombs were dropping all around them. As I said, no rhyme or reason. They behaved outside their normally rational day-to-day life, confounding even themselves. It's only after such irrational, intense actions that the process begins in coping with the possible outcomes, that is, their marital status, current relationships, children and even sexual health issues. So as a human race, we need to understand that some events and reactions are often experienced outside normal parameters and both males and females are at risk of stepping over the invisible line during times of extreme duress. Less judgment, more acceptance and support is needed for such people.

Another peculiar body reaction occurs when a male breaks his hip. Ambulance officers and medical personnel report with every male hip that is broken there is an erection. This situation is so common, personnel will automatically treat it as such when transporting the man to the hospital. So ponder that anomaly. If you think men are in control of their erections and are sick individuals because it rises to all sorts of occasions, then you just might have to rethink that idea. Recognize that men can become just as frustrated and embarrassed by their out-of-control penile behavior.

Lack of Public Affection

A partner might exhibit a high tendency to be affectionate and always show their feelings in a readable and outward manner. There is no mistaking the affection or accepting it at a heart level unless you function in the opposite. An unaffectionate person due to past events might experience this as smothering and it causes them to feel locked in. The affectionate person, on the other hand, feels rejected, pushed aside and dismissed. An inner dialogue of anxiety might activate crippling fights or cause a hasty hurt-filled retreat, which then simmers for months or years.

There is only so much rejection a person can take, unless they've been conditioned at a young age to accept this. So the unaffectionate person might have memories of parents who did not fight, so everything was calm, but the parents kept their loving embraces private, away from the child. A child might then grow up believing that public affection is not appropriate or normal. So they do not automatically act like this.

If a man doesn't show affection in public, but waits for the bedroom then gets down to business, he could be set up for a fall as his partner is desperately seeking more affection and foreplay from him. He has no love language to support her needs. The transition might be slow, and he will need to be gently taught without accusations of purposeful rejection.

However, if you as a partner have been brought up feeling affectionate as a child, but with every attempt to demonstrate affection you were swiped aside all the time, then you might have been trained to believe that you are not good enough. So when an unaffectionate partner reinforces your internal fears, you will react with paranoia and hurt. This could have you huddling in the corner of the bed, weeping yourself quietly to sleep, and daily anguishing about those memories. It makes it much harder to attempt connection in fear of rejection and being emotionally abandoned to a state of loneliness. This is definitely not the correct ingredient for dramatic and passionate lovemaking.

When I was 19 years old, I ended up living with a woman who had a gay son. I asked her son if he'd ever tried having sex with women. He replied that, yes, he had a girlfriend once, but she showed him no affection, just like the memories of his mother. He said that's when he realized that he was attracted to men, because they shared the same gender so obviously they shared the same emotional needs and expression. Women were not for him, because they were not capable of deep loving and emotionalism.

At the time of him expressing this, I was aware that he was already realizing that his male partner also exhibited the same unemotional tendencies. So his gay parameters of thinking were being challenged, and he was facing the prospect that he might have been wrong. He was beginning to delve into his subconscious language and internal drivers, looking for the possible causes of why he thought the way he did in relation to his upbringing and chosen sexual identification.

This gives us all great pause to look deep into our own pasts and see if we have hidden contributors that affect how we love and communicate with others.

Emotions, a Sign of Weakness

Many generations past, boys were ridiculed by their fathers for having a strong outpouring of emotions and were especially considered weak if they cried. Thankfully, this stance of conditioning is softening in Western culture, but it is still strong in Asia, Africa and Arabic nations. Men do not cry. A boy child learns young to not talk about feelings, because they might cry when they do and subsequently get punished for it. The way to solve the emotional situation is to bury it under lots of practical events. Keep busy, keep going and don't give yourself time to think and feel. Also parents would support a young child and the developing man by showing him how to solve the problem, tell him to take action and then work and distract himself more.

So a boy conditioned at a young age will think that to be a real man and accepted into a man-world, there is an unsaid entry criterion: men do not cry. And if you're upset, keep busy. Bury it. The boy swallows all his natural feelings and might also walk the planet believing he's not good enough to be heard. So in later years, he never expresses his real nature. This causes a partner to experience him as closed and not expressive. More accusations can come. If the woman is expressive, she'll be deemed irrational, hysterical and her partner will suggest she just get on with it, work harder and she'll feel better.

Well now, this is a funny thing. The man releases his pent-up stress and emotion with sex, so as he tries to help his hysterical partner, he offers her the best solution possible—great sex with him. Yep. He's sure that this will make her feel so much better, and he honestly believes he's helping, when all he can focus on is his instant solution—sex. I'm sorry, guys. If you think this is a good solution, then think again! You will totally flabbergast and anger a woman if you offer your services like that. She'll be confounded by your audacity to dare to offer it. She'll also be convinced that you are one selfish son-of-a-bitch. The truth is you were trying to make her feel better.

It's a bit like a child handing a parent a teddy or a doll to cuddle when they seem upset. It's simplistic and comes from the right intention from the heart, so ladies, you also need to think deeper about your partner's real intentions before taking offense and becoming even angrier. Laugh a little to lighten the load.

Low Body Image

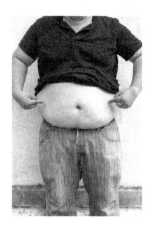

Physical Anatomy

Low body image is the single most common issue people face when it comes to intimacy. Men and women around the globe, face varying degrees of paranoia at how their bodies present to society and especially in relation to attracting the opposite sex and remaining attractive. Issues of weight, stretch marks, birthmarks, scarring, limb deformities, size, shape and contours of sexual organs enters the mind game that wraps itself insidiously within the intimacy sector of relationships.

As society urges people to compare themselves to one another and to media images, the psychological hurdle only gets bigger. How on earth does anyone feel good about themselves and their nakedness after the constant onslaught of public images? Well, the truth is, society is suffering badly, and I see daily the most exquisite beautiful young people seeking counseling and support for their total lack of love for their youthful bodies and the psychosis of self-reprimand and negative talk that finds its way into everyone's bedrooms.

Of course, it's not just the young who feel this way. Most commonly, it's the low self-image after having children, with issues of vaginal changes, sagging breasts, weight gain, and stretch marks. The women are left with all the changes as they gift new life, yet the man is left untouched. The women secretly carry real fears that they will no longer remain attractive to their partner. This fear is intensified when they catch the roving eye of their man looking at youthful pre-birth bodies as they face their own drastically lowered libido. A woman at this time feels vulnerable. She needs more loving attention and reassurance than at any other time.

To morph from being a childless woman with abundant energy, light-heartedness and often a much higher sex drive, into a consumed, exhausted and loveless female who feels the weight of responsibility on her shoulders, is a shocking betrayal of her idea of life's grand promises. Confidence to rip one's clothes off and stand naked in front of a partner might become that much harder if a lot of admiration and reassurance is not given. This lack of confidence is further fueled if there are layers of subconscious damage from early childhood sitting under the surface. Any event or action that makes the mind face possible feelings of inadequacy from earlier times will find a fertile environment to now enact paranoia.

Let us not forget men in this equation for they too can suffer terribly with lowered confidence if their body becomes sick, overweight, maimed or badly scarred.

Genital Anatomy

There seems to be an increase in paranoia around how the sexual organs look to our partner. In the past men had to face their body image by comparing themselves to other men when viewing their father or family relatives, in the public toilet urinals or sporting clubrooms. Men's penises hang externally and are therefore not hidden from the eye. This has meant men have faced the issue of penile comparison throughout history and is the cause behind many jokes and innuendo. Behind the brevity of such locker room talk men can still feel quite challenged and fearful about how they measure up in the eyes of their female partners especially in the early dating days. Insecurity can find it's way into the bedroom.

Women on the other hand have been left totally in the dark in relation to genital comparison with other females until recently with the advent of easy access pornography. Very rare would it be that females would actually see the female genitalia of their vulva let alone that of other women as its so well hidden by its anatomical position and in the past pubic hair has further obscured the view. These days paranoia on how their vulva looks has become so mind consuming that young women even in their teens are seeking out labiaplasty in an attempt to look more like the x-rated magazines or screen models they now see. We are witnessing a new low when it comes to self image among the young due to the explosion of pornography making it so much easier for male and females to view other people's genitals and make personal comparison.

As a society we do not usually comment when making love about another people's shape, size or color of their genitalia. These days that is changing along with grooming expectations. A new anxiety is pervading the minds of both genders creating alarming levels of suffering and impacting the confidence in relationships. Increased reassurance is vital to help sooth the way for relaxed loving.

Ladies: Many countries have media laws preventing vulva images to be shown in their honesty and are photo-shopped. Please keep in mind, research shows men love vaginas in all shapes and sizes! If they didn't, pornography and magazines would fizzle out.

Lights On, Lights Off

Are you a "lights on" or "lights off" lover? Do you like your body enough to let your partner see your beautiful, natural nakedness? Do you feel shame about yourself or worried he or she will judge you?

Men and women feel uneasiness at times if they stand or lay down naked in full view of their partner. Their mind is conjuring all manner of possible rejection scenarios or personal judgment placed on them when being intently looked at by another. Also in the middle of trying to enjoy the moment of loving early foreplay, this can really interfere in their minds. There are those people who love the openness of exchange and others who freak out and wither inside. The ones who wither inside will maneuver in any way possible to get to the light switch and turn off the intensity. It's the only way they can go on and half relax to be able to have any enjoyment in the sexual act.

So where does the paranoia come from? There are times in early life and natural nakedness that parents might act in alarmed ways and take swift actions and strong words to cover up an innocent child's body or genitalia. Depending on the emotional intensity of the moment, children might take on feelings and beliefs that their bodies are shameful, ugly, and too dirty for others outside the family to look at. Words from parents damage—once said, the damage is done. This is also true of other children, schoolteachers, and any people of influence outside the family home.

If belief systems such as this become locked within the subconscious mind, they will ultimately resurface later and often it's in a relationship. So remaining clothed until the last minute before sex or turning the light off is a usual response. Here again, sexual abuse also rages its negative psychological effect.

If people feel complete shame and dirty by an event, then any intimate act later will potentially bring the shame feelings on and they'll want to hide in the darkness. Deep down, they fear that the lights turned on will reveal what they did as a child. They blame and shame themselves for the sexual abuse.

I'm here to tell you that it's possible to heal from these events and begin a journey of loving intimacy and accepting your body. You can peel back the layers of negative words and behaviors that parents and other abusers have instilled in you. It takes courage, but it is possible.

Clothes Off, Socks On

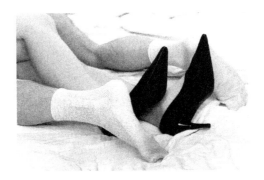

What is it with men being naked but leaving their socks on? Are they ready to take a run straight after sex? Men, you need to know it's a turn-off for most women. Usually it takes away from the beautiful lines of a naked body and makes a woman feel that you're not completely there with her in the moment. You are still on the run. So take them off.

Of course, everyone has their personal preference about sexuality and individual fantasies, but leaving socks on does not come up often as a female fantasy! Sadly, it's more common that women don't like to uncover their bodies to their partner. They leave their clothes on until the last minute as they climb into bed. They're less likely to disrobe all over the house, share the enjoyment of a shower, bath or skinny-dipping together. So many elements of fun, laughter and togetherness that create memories throughout a lifetime are left untouched. If the woman does not unclothe for the man to see her, the visual male has a lessened sexual life due to the visual deprivation. He might still have fulfilled sex, but his visual centers, where fantasies and memories are kept, have been left unfulfilled.

For all these different scenarios, the question begs to be answered—what is motivating people's actions, behaviors and reactions? How can one person love her body being looked at and another person squirms away from exploring eyes? The truth lays in the psychology of a person being damaged in early life. If those issues become dominant, then experiencing life to the fullest will be diminished and the full joys of love, intimacy and sex can be sorely tested. These issues magnify and cause hypersensitivity in relation to criticism, both obvious and perceived.

Hypersensitivity

Relationships of all kinds, in all walks of life, have a unique capacity to go around in circles. Psychological issues arise from the subconscious from years gone past into the conscious and are translated into the events in the now. So when we talk and express ourselves, we're not only talking about thoughts and feelings of the now, but also expressing our deeper feelings of the past that have been influencing us to the present moment.

Now, this is where conducting a relationship becomes really tricky. As a woman, you might be trying to talk to your partner about how he ignores you all the time. The truth is he might only switch off and ignore you at specific times and, on average, only about 40 percent of the time. Your exaggeration stems from your dad who was always busy working, then watching TV and not listening to your child-like stories. This totaled 40 percent of the time in your childhood memories of experience.

So the two males you love the most, your dad and your partner, are ignoring you with a combined total of 80 percent lack of attention. That's huge and hurtful, and so your equal reaction matches that at 80 percent. Then add an extra 10 percent of magnified reaction because, as in life, we increase the story and we increase the memories. So, of course, the subsequent effect of this is your own increased reaction against the male for what he has said and what he has done. Then through that increased reaction and your perception being quite unfair and imbalanced, you will attack your partner, which then creates damage and scar tissue to his psychological being. Worse still, your reaction triggers his personal early patterning about being falsely accused. He gets his back up and adds more fuel to the fire and the self-perpetuating cycle begins.

Self-Perpetuating Relationship Cycle

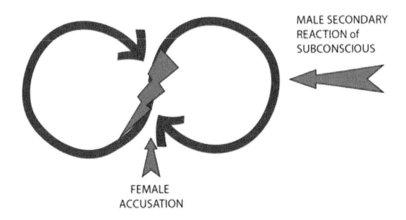

SELF PERPETUATING RELATIONSHIP CYCLE

MALE SECONDARY REACTION of SUBCONSCIOUS

FEMALE ACCUSATION

If we don't understand the basic fundamental elements of psychology, then any attempts at balanced relationships are doomed. The depth of one's self is junk-filled redundant thought processes, beliefs and programs and emotional conditioning that must be deprogrammed before balance can arrive in any relationship with others.

Don't try to fix your parental and childhood issues by using your partner as a battering ram. Become aware of the truth behind a partner's actions and behavior compared to your reactions to past family issues, and don't pollute one with the other. Keep them separate. Delve deep and find true honesty with oneself.

If blaming another helps you to feel power, then find out why and when you feel powerless. If being a victim, find out how being a victim and having sympathy helped you feel loved and secure. If you attack others to make you always feel right and in control, find out why you have felt powerless and full of fear. If you have the courage to explore this truth about yourself, then you'll become a better and more-balanced person in all of your life dealings. Better still, those people you love will see a realistic version of you and will love you for who you are and not what you are.

Sex, Anxiety and Secrets in Relationships

Men and women are plagued by anxiety about their sex lives. Negative thoughts, anxieties and fears eat into every part of their daily routines, work lives and careers. When they are with a partner, they know they will have to face, at some stage, their fears and anxieties head on. They know, sooner or later, it will be asked of them to allow sexual contact to keep the relationship on an even keel. Dread can be a partner to these events when it really should be sacred.

For men and woman to get to such a point of feeling twisted and contorted about when, where and how they will have to make love when they really are not wanting to, can be soul destroying. The usual formula that women use to help themselves is by talking to friends, mothers or sisters, but in the very private arena of coupling it does not usually happen. They fake happiness; they carry the burden of private events that have occurred in the bedroom. They harbor such tragic stories that need healing support and insight to give them the power to ask for something different out of life. Or even to speak up and say no.

When deep, open and frank discussions with friends don't happen, most women feel isolated. Women speak about so many other events in their life openly, but to speak truthfully of their sex life is like admitting a deep failure and vulnerability they don't want to show anyone. It is deeply personal. They might make jokes about their partner but don't usually go into extreme detail, because it's personal and they don't want the public to belittle or make light of the closest physical interaction two people can have.

Men also have their own inadequacies with open talking among friends. If they talk to women, then they begin to feel emotionally open and think that these pleasant feelings might need to be expressed in a sexual way. This only complicates the opportunity to open up and so they eventually clam up again. They become paralyzed within themselves to show weakness to their fellow humans, being fearful that it shows their inability to keep on top of the game. They too become isolated, withdrawn and anxious.

I have been blessed with the courage of so many men and women who have spoken with me and opened up with their deepest secrets and concerns. I have carried their pain and stories with me, holding them so they might carry on with their lives knowing that one person on the planet knows the truth of who they are, who they have become and why they think and feel the way they do. To be a counselor has been the greatest honor, and I want to share some of the basic story lines they have shared with me so if there are other women or men out there with similar experiences, then you know you are not alone. These basic stories might give you the courage to seek extra help and support from health professionals.

Violence in the Bedroom

It is a sad fact that when we couple with someone, we don't really know how they will treat our most vulnerable self, the sexual side of our nature and our naked truth.

A partner who looks great, successful, connected, together, popular and charismatic might well indeed have serious low self-esteem issues and these can arise hidden from public view and played out in the bedroom. Violence, jealousy, accusations, coerced sexual acts and even rape in the marriage all occur behind closed doors. I have listened to the most beautiful, kind, caring women, successful, normal day-to-day women, who all harbor tormented secrets, such as these, with huge psychological impact often resulting in alcohol addiction, self-harm and terminal disease.

He seems like a wonderful man until he drinks too much, comes home and rapes his wife in the room next to his sleeping, or so he thought, daughters. Struggling whimpers escape as the mother tries to keep this knowledge from her children.

Let it be known that men also suffer violence perpetrated upon them by female partners. I spent some time on a National Crisis phone line and I often heard stories where the man was the victim of continual physical abuse. So let's dispel the myth that it's only females that suffer at the hand of their male partners. Abuse comes in many forms, mental, emotional, physical and financial.

For the focus of this book I deal essentially with the physical violence but all forms of abuse will create a wave of distress that will be played out in the bedroom. It would take a completely separate book to deal with the intense nature of domestic violence and abuse within relationships to give the topic justice.

Role Playing and Cross Dressing

Women are totally confused and mystified as to why a man wants to wear her clothes or panties and parade in them, thinking she will be turned on by such sights. She is then expected, once he is turned on by his actions, to behave sexually aroused yet within the core of her being, she wants to vomit. The reaction might be quite different if a partner is role-playing and dressing up in an outfit. There is potential for some light-hearted fun and laughter. Everyone loves light heartedness however if the role- playing becomes sadistic and hurtful and only one person of this activity is enjoying themselves, then a recipe for disaster is created.

Erotic Clothes and Sex Toys

Some men demand to have a woman wear specific clothing or use sex toys, as it is the only way the man can be visually turned on. This makes some woman feel ugly, have no confidence in her own appeal and feel like just a piece of flesh for the man to insert himself into.

With same-sex couples, one partner might pressure the other partner to try hardcore styles of sex that might be considered normal within some circles. This causes quite a bit of anxiety, as they do not wish to cause problems by saying an outright NO.

Degrading Sexual Talk and Demoralizing Body Image

Women trying to escape intimacy might deploy an arsenal of ferocious negative talk to the man, hoping he will not approach them with sexual advances. He feels torn, shredded, gutted and becomes isolated. This can happen on a daily basis, rather than the women learning the tools to speak up about her fears. Two people end up being damaged and unsupported.

Men on the other hand may use a whole collection of words and suggestions relating to the females sex appeal or lack there of due to body changes or through constant comparisons to past lovers.

Teenagers and Hardcore Sex and Threesomes

Teenagers and young adults are constantly feeling the pressure to participate in hardcore sex acts as seen on porn sites. Young men and women now believe that the images and video footage so easily accessed are the normal way to experience intimacy. Has society gone too far? The stories I am being told in my clinic and backed by reports from other practitioners are saying, "Yes, society has a newfound struggle with inadvertent sexual abuse within young developing relationships."

There are so many more stories that all end up in a terrible silent depression.

Celia Fuller

{ 8 }
Seek Support –
Replace Apathy With Action

It is my greatest hope that this book will take you a long way in understanding yourself and your partner and answering so many of the frustrations you face. However, there might need to be a more serious look at some of the deeper issues that might be arising within the relationship for long-term success.

There are the usual therapies that most people know about and often use. The obvious one is going to a doctor and proclaiming your woes. Here is a humorous story of how past doctors dealt with female emotions and ended up inventing the vibrator as the solution.

Story

In our not-that-distant history, if a woman complained about her issues involving sexuality and home life concerns, it was called female hysteria. In 1734 in France, one of the earliest known vibrators was invented as a means to relieve doctors of the tedious task of manipulating the vulva until the female had a "hysterical paroxysm" (orgasm), which then relieved some of her worst symptoms for a time. When doing manual masturbation, they did not even recognize it as a sexual act, but saw it as a physical disjointed manipulation that took a long time to actually have physical success.

The invention of the vibrator came about to relieve the doctors of their repetitive strain injuries and wasted clinical hours. For an amusing rendition of a later invention of the vibrator, watch the movie *Hysteria*, as it's based on historical events and is funny. It's even a good one for opening up those delicate conversations at home.

Back then, if the doctor's manual manipulation did not work to relieve the woman, then the next stage of therapy was often a hysterectomy, as it was said that it would be the cure because the woman was obviously hysterical. When a woman entered menopause age and started speaking up for herself and becoming slightly agitated, then she would be deemed to have lost her marbles and needed respite or permanent incarceration into a nut house, sorry sanitarium.

This is just a gentle reminder that those unusual attitudes were not that long ago and as a society, we have really advanced in the knowledge of men's and women's sexuality. Having said that, there are still many people scattered around the globe who remain living their lives without this information and make rash assumptions about the nature of illness that besieges a woman's mind and makes her act in a manner deemed erratic and unstable.

So in this modern age, when you go to a doctor, you will more often than not be told you are depressed and fed a tablet to make you get better, thus suppressing for a time the core problem. If you are lucky, you will be referred to a psychologist or psychiatrist before taking medication to find out what lies behind all the erratic emotional states. At the very least, they might refer you to a local counselor. They are usually hesitant to do this, because they do not have the same level of training in their view as the other medical health professionals who are closer to their own standing.

Some people, especially men, dodge any mention of counseling if they possibly can. They believe it shows a certain type of weakness within a person's character. Now I know a lot of people who go to counseling but spend hours talking week after week but never feeling like they are getting anywhere. They do gain some insight, but it does not give great power to make the changes they really need at a deeper level. They change the external behavior, but don't really dig deeper to find the subconscious behaviors and patterns that might be triggering them.

Other people seek the cheaper alternative route of counseling by bestowing the hairdresser, massage therapist, natural therapist, barperson, secretary, and their gym trainer with all manner of their life stories. They have talked and made themselves feel better for a time but eventually they go full circle and again need debriefing.

There Is Another Way—Alternative Solutions

There are so many alternative therapies, often thought of as quackery, but in our enlightened modern world, we have more knowledge of the brain and we better understand the actions of the subconscious and neural networking. This is changing our understanding of reality and human behavior.

Science is reluctantly accepting these alternative therapies that have been around for thousands of years, because of the latest leaps in research. At times, they are even accelerating the success stories by weaving scientific language around ideas that have been understood by medicine men in cultures and continents throughout the world. These plentiful therapies are proving to be effective in unearthing the true issues behind the complex emotional, mental and sexual complaints that couples might have.

I will provide a partial list for you, but it does not cover them all.

Exercise

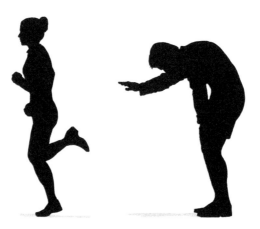

Most people think exercise is a sport, but, in fact, it really is a deep therapy for the body. The body is meant to move, to hunt, to gather, to awaken intelligence through muscle memory. A child does not learn how to manage itself in the world without movement being the first and foremost activity for survival and cognitive skill development. This essential life requirement has not changed since the dawn of time. We need to move! When a level of fitness is experienced, it switches on the pleasure hormones of the brain, thus uplifting our mood and our external senses.

Great athletes and those who lose significant weight by getting their bodies moving often experience huge increases of sexual energy. The support crew for the Olympics held in Australia in 2000 was shocked at how often the condom vending machine in the athlete's village emptied after major events were finished. This gives rise to the idea of oversexed people or certainly ones who had withheld for some time before their events, only to unleash their full power afterward. So get your body moving! Any exercise is good exercise and it does not have to be costly.

Yoga, Thai Chi, Qi Gong

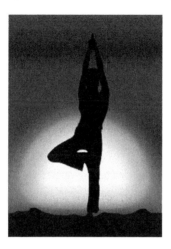

Yoga, Thai Chi, Qi Gong and water aerobics are all calm, controlled slow-moving exercises that can be adapted for the elderly or anyone with injuries or impediments of any kind. I have even seen a remarkable YouTube video of army paratrooper Arthur Boorman, who was relegated for 15 years to walking with sticks. He decided he wanted change in his life. He found a trainer who believed in him and he began training and then began with the easiest and most gentle yoga movements. During the course of six months, he transformed himself. He could run, lost considerable weight, his sexual drive picked up and he felt fantastic. He actually looked fantastic. What struck me the most was that he never gave up, even when he fell to the floor when trying standing yoga postures.

When we see other people fulfilling their goals, then it gives us the permission to try. This might not fix your sex life, but you might just feel fabulous, look fabulous and enjoy your sexless life and revitalized body that much more.

Mindfulness Meditation

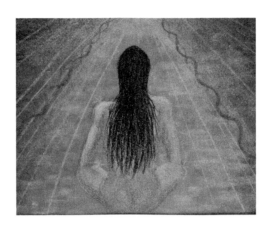

I have been practicing and teaching meditation for 25 years and found it to be the ultimate in stress reduction. What is meditation, you might ask? It is the disciplined art of being aware of your mind while you observe the sensations of the inflow and outflow of breath. Now some people observe the breath filling up their abdomen and then observe the sensation and motion as the abdomen deflates. Other people use another method of watching the breath coming in and out of the nasal passages. Both approaches work. It is a merely a matter of choice and you can also combine the two processes. When you first start, begin with the abdomen approach. Then as you become comfortable with this, you bring your attention higher up to the nasal passages.

This focalized attention of breath watching, gradually has the effect of quieting your daily rambling busy thoughts. Our thoughts stimulate reactions, and if we are not careful, then our thoughts are filled with fear and anxiety, which can stir up a hornet's nest of emotion for us. This often triggers a physical reaction by using unmonitored words in response to a situation. Chaos follows.

The quietness attained in meditation allows space for a truthful evaluation of your own value system and personal perspective on life events. There is an intensified sensation of observing your thoughts and realizing how they contribute to relationship inter-action and possible antagonistic stimulus. Meditation has been around for thousands of years and is considered an intricate part of Eastern culture. It is often wrongly associated with only reli-gious activity.

In the modern era with the advent of brain scans, CAT scans, ECGs and EEGs, more research has been revealing the great and varied changes that meditation can have on the mind and body. It is definitely known to lessen the stress responses and give the per-son a deeper sense of calm and clarity. Through the mind calm-ing, a person will feel more rested with the potential of increased creative thoughts, inspiration and problem solving. It is an essen-tial, simple tool that should be added to your life.

For me, meditation increased my intuition. This helped me to be aware of my own feelings and reactions around sexuality and how I was processing all the convoluted changes that happen to the body after children with a maturing relationship. It taught me to become brutally honest with my feelings and behaviors, so I could make more positive choices.

The years of practice also sensitized my persona to hear the unsaid words and thoughts of clients. I was able to formulate the correct questions to help guide them into opening up with their stories that they would have otherwise held onto, not sure if they wanted to tell me for fear of uncovering weakness and vulnerabil-ity. Essentially, I believe I short tracked otherwise potential long counseling sessions that would normally take a therapist many visits to uncover. Some of the people left unburdened after one session.

Blueprint Healing— An Energetic Healing Therapy

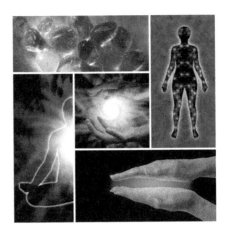

As a spiritual teacher and practitioner, I use traditional methods of counseling and an alternative form of healing within my clinic and across the world through phone calls and Skype sessions. For over twenty years, I have been sharing my gift with others and facilitating incredible change in people's lives, often after only one session. The results never cease to amaze me.

Working with the psychology of the person, I fast track the sessions by using my intuitive skills to locate the core event when a traumatic experience or programmed belief system became locked within the subconscious mind. This event becomes the hidden saboteur to your success in dealing with life, love, work, career, family and your own mental and emotional processing. Through the unique blueprint healing modality I have formulated, once the origin of an issue is detected, with your permission I send threads of energy through time and space to your past, unlocking and unwinding the negatives effects. This process is essentially like placing an updated version of software and rebooting your system. You are an active participant in this process.

I can say that many people have enjoyed enormous reboots

directly to their sex lives. For those who have taken a little more time, because of their complex psychological makeup, together we have found that when they move through their emotional and mental issues that have accumulated throughout their lifetimes, it is amazing how issues of not speaking up, low self-worth, guilt, shame and self-punishment can be resolved through this system. Thousands have commented that it has helped them communicate more openly and with confidence with their partner and from there, they have enjoyed a deeper sense of intimacy and personal empowerment.

www.wholistic-lifestyles.com.au

Hypnotherapy

Hypnotherapy, often understood as a stand-alone therapy, is in fact a combination of many therapies all used by the therapist and coined into one word. Other therapies associated with the term hypnotherapy are regression therapy, suggestion therapy and Neuro-Linguistic Programming (NLP).

Popular belief has it that a hypnotherapist can control your mind, but, in fact, the opposite is true. In any one session, the participant has to give permission and be ready to accept the process, otherwise it is useless. A few sessions are required at first to create a familiar environment and to build an effective rapport between the therapist and the client. Then the real work can begin.

Regression therapy is a process where the participant, through a relaxed mind, can be gently guided through time to past events causing the behavior, neurosis, hidden trauma and habits that might be dictating unusual or reactive responses within a person's life. This could be a powerful tool to unearth reasons behind some of the emotional responses being experienced within relationships. It is done safely without reliving the events, but looks at the events as though through a window as an observer.

Suggestion therapy is a technique that can be used without regression therapy. The therapist, through talking, can identify a habitual pattern that you would like to change. With the support of the therapist, you will find the correct words and approach required to present the subconscious mind with specific suggestion language to make changes in future behavior and choices in your life.

Neuro-Linguistic Programming is the art of using specific language that the subconscious instantly relates to and will activate the positive affirmed visualizations that are mentioned while in the relaxed hypnotic trance state.

Naturopaths, Herbalists, Homeopaths

These health professionals can use a myriad of vitamins, minerals, herbs and homeopathic remedies to bring an internal physiological change in the body. Many people think they are depressed and begin to blame situations in the home, rather than suspecting underlying health conditions that could be easily remedied with simple inquiry, not needing the full force of the medical field.

Many vitamin and mineral imbalances can trigger effects within the hormonal system and brain processing capabilities. Herbs can strengthen and tone internal organs, increasing their output and increasing one's sense of vitality and well-being. There are even some herbal products that can indeed increase, to a degree, libido. They have nothing to do with killing animals for an aphrodisiac.

Chiropractic, Osteopathic, Massage

These therapies are all manual in nature and have their own health-giving purpose for the body. Chiropractic and osteopathic treatments release trapped or contorted spinal nerves within the spine, which are radiating into the extremities of the body. These contortions can occur even by minor degrees through muscle spasm or injury. The nerves feeding through the spine are responsible for the commands to the rest of the body through constant impulses. These might become impeded, causing a widespread variety of body sensations, pain and chemical hormonal regulatory imbalances.

It is well known that lower back injuries can directly affect sexual function in both male and females. The obvious external hint of this is impotence in men. Many times a chiropractor or osteopath has been able to release the affected nerves and released the mental burden a man carries when afflicted in this manner.

Let's not discount the amazing effects that massage can bring. Deep penetrating massage can facilitate great changes in muscle action, where spasms and incorrect tensions are causing the spine to distort. With a well-trained therapist who can incorporate massage and gentle stretching techniques, the body can begin regulating itself and the spine will make slow natural adjustments. There are many techniques within a therapist's tool chest to help improve health and vitality just by the use of safe human touch. It can help a person still feel connected to other humans and provide a window of time while dealing with the deeper complex nature of psychology or lack of communication that might be getting in the way of intimate relations.

Acupuncture and Bowen Therapy

Bowen Therapy is a gentle muscle manipulation technique, which acts directly with the nervous system and indirectly with the meridian system associated with the Eastern modality of acupuncture. There are amazing results that can be facilitated by both acupuncture and Bowen Therapy within the internal body systems, rhythms and the external extremities. Whenever there is increased health, there is a higher degree of emotional and mental coping with longed-for stress reduction. This helps a person process life in a much more balanced way.

Kinesiology

Kinesiology is a therapy that uses a specific method to test the different muscle strengths all over the body and provide feedback to the practitioner and client. The located imbalances in the body might be causing distress, pain or neuralgia. These weaknesses are then altered and strengthened with the client experiencing the lessening or eradication of uncomfortable symptoms. The therapy has developed into a more complex variety of therapies.

Emotional kinesiology uses the same technique to question the body's cellular memory bank. By specific questioning and testing, the practitioner can locate the origin of emotional trauma and beliefs that have settled into the body and the subconscious. The practitioners facilitate their techniques to release these memories, thus freeing a person from the trauma and gifting them relief from their inner anguish.

Australian Bush and Bach Flower Essences

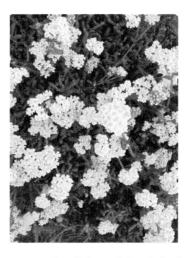

As far back as the 1930s, Dr. Edward Bach believed that physical illness originated in the emotional and mental imbalances within the person. He went on to develop a series of remedies based on flower essences to address these imbalances. His remedies proved to be a huge success, and people all over the world still use them with great effect. In Australia, there is another therapy inspired by his remedy model, Australian Bush Flower Essences. These were created by a fifth-generation naturopath, Ian White.

Both therapies create great changes in the psychological makeup of a person and effect positive change in their behaviors and reactions. Some of the remedies are specific for sexual issues.

Other Healing Practices

Faith Healing

It would be remiss of me not to mention the power of the church and its role in supporting congregation members. By the use of confessionals, churchgoers can release a lot of the burden of their lives onto someone else's shoulders, allowing them to keep moving forward. The priest is often used like a counselor in the confessional. There are also the Christian denominations that do fantastic hands-on healing and other vast networks of support that also facilitates great change for those with faith. I always recommend people go to practitioners who will support their personal belief systems and not take away from what they have as their foundation.

Reiki

Reiki is another energetic hands-on healing modality that transfers universal energy through the practitioner's body and energy system, gifting it to the client. It is relaxing, releases huge levels of stress and, for some people, it will lift the burden of emotional and mental issues.

In Summary

I apologize to all those in the community that I may not have represented fully with the ideas and explanations in this book. It is not my intention to cause offence to cultural or sexual persuasions of different groups. I can only hope that you may have gained some insights and converted my representations to meet your own needs.

The human psyche is multilayered and multifaceted. This book only scratches the surface of the complex nature of relationships and relating to one another. There is always room for improvement in any relationship and as we navigate our ways around each other let it be done with Loving Kindness, Compassion and Understanding.

Connect With Me

Help Me, Help Others

I love getting feedback from my readers and would really appreciate you taking a few minutes to post your comments or a brief review on my Amazon Page.

www.amazon.com/author/celiafuller

Also come join our Facebook community here: Facebook: Celia-Fuller-Inspirational-Speaker-Spiritual-Teacher

About Celia Fuller

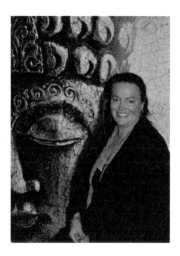

During the past two decades, Celia Fuller has been a partner with her husband in a natural therapies and counseling business, focusing on health and wellbeing for the mind, body and spirit.

Celia, through her **wholistic lifestyle consultancy** sessions and much sought-after speaking events has provided incredible **insight** to thousands of people's lives. She has given them the tools and knowledge to assist with reclaiming their personal power and walking them ever closer to their personal success. She helps break the invisible barriers that stand in the way of people reaching their full potential, rising through the corporate ladder or simply finding greater harmony in their life.

Companies and businesses have sought her counsel in relation to the purchase or sale of properties, business dealings, work dynamics of staff and client training. Individuals have sought her out for family issues, settlements, work situations, real estate and relationship issues. Her specialized sessions often incorporate the use of meditation for managing stress and spiritual philosophy to offer a broader view on life.

She has had the privilege and honor of listening to many private concerns of thousands of clients. Through their stories, she noted the repeat pattern of mind-consuming anxiety around sexual dynamics within their relationships, resulting in lowered expectation of fulfilling their dreams and passions. Depression, low performance in the work place, lack of focus, lack of Inspiration for life, work or business caused them to feel confused, baffled and erratic. For this reason, this book had to be written.

Helpful Links and Resources

Recommended Books

The Multi-Orgasmic Man: Sexual Secrets Every Man Should Know by Mantak Chia and Douglas Abrams

Australian Bush Flower Essences by Ian White

Men Are from Mars, Women Are from Venus: The Classic Guide to Understanding the Opposite Sex by John Gray

Websites

Kegel Pelvic Muscle Exercises:
www.mayoclinic.org
www.prevention.com

Explicit Sexual Instruction from a Woman's Point of View:
www.mytinysecrets.com

YouTube Videos

"Amazing Power of Yoga for Overall Health"
Arthur Boorman—Healed through Yoga:
http://www.youtube.com?watch?=9x9FSZJu448.

A Final Thank You…

**These inspirational people have inspired my own journey during the past years.
I now add my life work to theirs.**

Richard Branson—One of his first entrepreneurial efforts was to create a sexual health help line for the young. He did this at great risk of imprisonment, as it was illegal to refer so openly about sexual matters at that time in history. He believed in more awareness and openness about sexuality, as I do. He has continued to inspire people through his life choices and business philosophy of pursuing your dreams and great ideas and seeing where they take you.

Oprah Winfrey—A strong spokeswoman for women and exploring any avenue she could to help people come to understand themselves better. Through guest speakers, she addressed many of the phobias and attitudes that women hold hidden within themselves, desperate to be understood. She inspires through her own life journey in such a powerful way, not shying away from critics.

Deepak Chopra and Louise Hay—They have gifted the world a lifetime of knowledge and awareness, encouraging others to do the same. They have been forerunners in opening up discussions about the interconnected relationship between the mind, body and spirit and our interdependence to the world around us.

Dalai Lama—A strong, peaceful, figurehead in a world that often feels so chaotic. His continued efforts, even into his old age, never cease to encourage humankind to treat one another with loving kindness, compassion and understanding. He has given me the strength to share my wisdom and insight.